Thank you for your support.
Imelda xxx

DEDICATION

This book is dedicated to my friend and fellow photographer, Alison Craven who sadly lost her battle with cancer in March 2018.

I would like to thank my husband, Andy, my parents, family, friends and the photographic community for their unwavering love and support and also Russell, Lesley, Mr Dani and all the other doctors and nurses who have looked after me over the past year.

Finally I want to thank Donia, without whom this book would not have been possible and everybody who has participated in this project.

FOREWORD

New research estimates that one in two of us will be diagnosed with cancer at some stage in our lives. The good news is that survival rates are higher than ever before. Scientific research is progressing all the time with focus on effective treatments and minimising side effects, allowing patients to maintain a quality of life.

Despite the ongoing research, receiving a diagnosis is a scary time for both the patient and their family.

Award-winning photography fellow and author, Imelda Bell, experienced this fear of the unknown, when she heard the words "you almost certainly have breast cancer". As a portrait photographer, Imelda started to document her experience, not only in the form of a diary, but also in self-portraits, as she went through chemotherapy and radiotherapy. Soon she explored the emotions of other people going through cancer treatment, using her talent as a photographer to create compelling photographs illustrating the side effects and emotions, which accompany this disease. These powerful images became a project Imelda called "Faces of Cancer".

Whilst there is lots of medical information available, Imelda found that she needed to see things from a patient perspective, and this was relatively limited. By sharing her story and "Faces of Cancer" in her book, "Facing the Monster" Imelda shows that there is a whole range of emotions that accompany this awful disease. Yes, there are times of fear, anger, frustration and sadness, but there are also times of joy and love. Imelda's images speak without words, and I am drawn into the photographs, wanting to know more about the stories behind them. Imelda takes us through her experience with a mixture of seriousness and humour, giving people an idea of what they might face if the monster calls on them.

This book is a wonderful study in portrait photography, depicting human emotions, as well as a personal story of triumph over adversity.

Imelda has faced the monster head on and while continuing to fight, she has turned a negative into a positive, which she hopes will inspire and comfort others.

CONTENTS

INTRODUCTION

My name is Imelda Bell, and in December 2017, I was diagnosed with Breast Cancer. I will never forget the words: "You almost certainly have cancer," and the frenzy of tests and biopsies that followed. The scariest thing was wondering what the future holds.

I am a photographer, and I have found it very therapeutic taking self-portraits depicting the emotions and side effects I have experienced. I started to take photos of other people with cancer, and "Faces of Cancer" was born.

It struck me how often people expect cancer patients to retreat into a miserable haze. Yes, there are dark days but the emotions that accompany this journey are varied, and it is a roller coaster with lots of positives as well as negatives.

Twenty of the images formed a panel, which saw me awarded a Fellowship with the Master Photographers Association. On Sunday the 7th October 2018, this went on to be awarded the Best Fellowship Panel of 2018.

The chairman of the MPA commented, "You have now achieved the greatest accolade possible to any photographer, the BEST Fellowship panel of the year, that stands head and shoulders above anything else you will ever do (except beating the big C). You are now standing at the very top, and your future is to help pull others up behind you. You cannot go higher with other little insignificant awards; you can only strive to improve and inspire others…"

That is what I want to do with "Faces of Cancer." To inspire not only other photographers but to help people affected by Cancer, through my imagery, to see that we can continue to live and enjoy life, and although there are scary and dark times, there are also times of happiness, tremendous love and laughter.

The aim of my series of images (of which there are now over 60, including about 40 self-portraits) is to help people to see that there is still life with cancer, even if it is terminal.

Sadly, on the evening of Monday the 8th of October, a day after I was presented with the award, one of the people in my panel, Scott Anderson, passed away. Scott was very proud to appear in this body of work, and I am honoured to have got to know him.

I want to dedicate my win to Scott, and I hope that his portrait, along with the others I have created, will help people throughout the world to deal with cancer. In memory of Scott, I am hoping to get these photos out to as many people as possible, to be displayed and exhibited where they will reach those who need to see them.

A CANCER DIARY

8 DECEMBER 2017

Lying in bed this morning, I rolled over and felt a tightening in my right breast. I'd been aware of a denser area on my breast for about six months, but I'd never felt a lump before. As my fingers rolled over the area, there was a definite lump I didn't notice before. I got up, showered, and checked the area several more times before convincing myself it was definitely something worth mentioning to my GP. I called the doctor's surgery to try and get an appointment. They were fully booked, so I explained to the receptionist why I needed to see someone, and she gave me a telephone appointment.

My GP called me back a short while later and told me to come in and see him later today. He examined me and felt the lump, and to be safe, he referred me to a consultant at the hospital to have it double-checked. As we pay for private healthcare insurance, I was referred very quickly, and my appointment is in just four days.

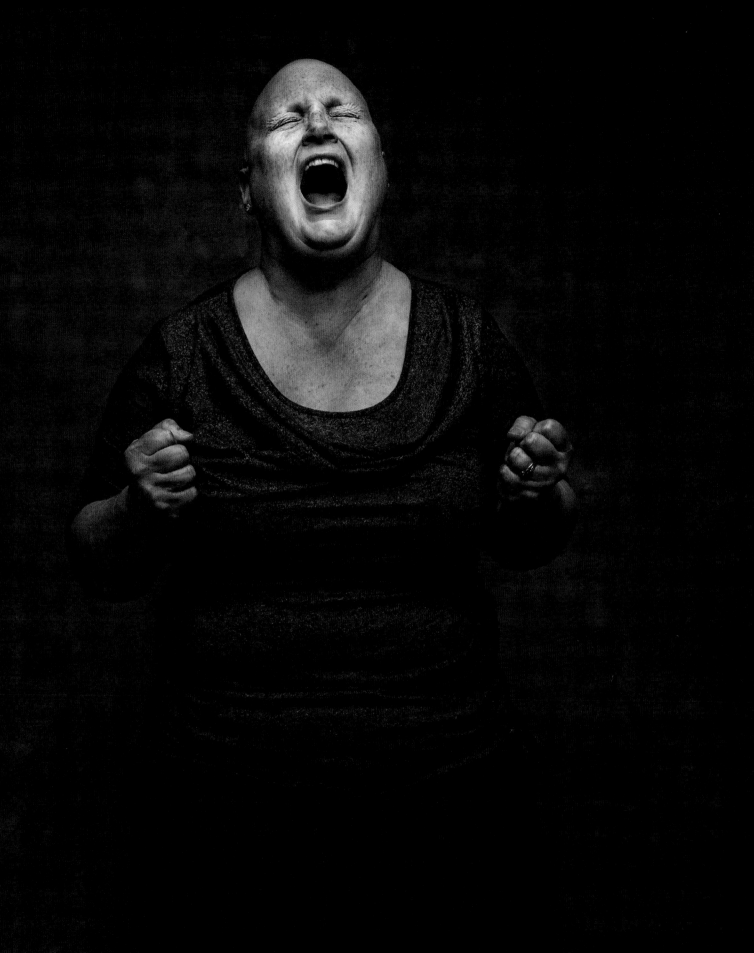

12 DECEMBER 2017

Confident that everything would be okay, I went to my appointment at the breast clinic on my own. My husband, Andy, had a late work meeting, so I said I would be fine. I arrived at the hospital and filled in a pile of forms before going through to see the consultant breast surgeon. We had a chat and he examined me, and I was sent for a mammogram and an ultrasound. I'd never had a mammogram before, as it is only a routine procedure in women over 50 years in the area where I live.

I had to undress and stand in front of the machine while the mammographer lifted my breast onto one of the Perspex plates. She squashed my breast as flat as it would go between the plates, while I stood there, dead-still on tiptoes with my arm held up, while they took the images. It was more uncomfortable than sore but was nothing to worry about. The process was then repeated at a different angle and on the other side. I didn't know what I was looking at, but I had a glance at the images while I redressed. The main thing I noticed were the blood vessels.

After the mammogram, I went straight to ultrasound, where I lay on the bed, stripped again to the waist (There is a theme going here!). Gel was applied, and the breast was scanned. The radiographer measured the mass and then took a sample for biopsy, which I took to be routine. First, injecting local anaesthetic near my nipple numbed the area, and then once it was numb, she inserted a spring-loaded needle, which took the sample. A few samples were taken, and I was escorted back to see the breast surgeon. I sat down and was taken over the findings of the scans.

"So, you've had a biopsy," said the consultant, and there is an area of DCIS (ductal carcinoma in situ)."

He went on to explain that this is an early form of breast cancer and showed up as an area with calcification. It made me chuckle to myself as he drew a pair of breasts to illustrate what he was saying. I suddenly had visions of him as a schoolboy drawing boobs on his textbooks — not a skill you ever think will come in handy as an adult!

Just think; breast surgeons go from being schoolboys doodling boobs on books, to drawing diagrams of boobs to explain things to patients, to actually drawing on real boobs on the morning of surgery!

I don't think I fully understood what he was saying until he then said the words you don't ever imagine you will hear, "You almost certainly have cancer!"

The rest of the appointment was a bit of a blur, but I remember getting emotional and fighting back tears at one point. The breast care nurse was very supportive and caring towards me, which really helped at this difficult time. Further tests were arranged, and another appointment was made for next week. I walked down the corridor towards the car in disbelief. I called Andy, and he rushed home to me on the next train.

13 DECEMBER 2017

Andy took the day off work so we could just spend some time together absorbing the news. We had a lovely brunch at a local farm shop, and my consultant called me while we were there. He said he doesn't normally call patients the day after an appointment, but I looked so shell-shocked and was all alone, so he wanted to make sure I was okay and to see if I had any questions. I was really touched by the fact that he cared enough to call me when he didn't have to.

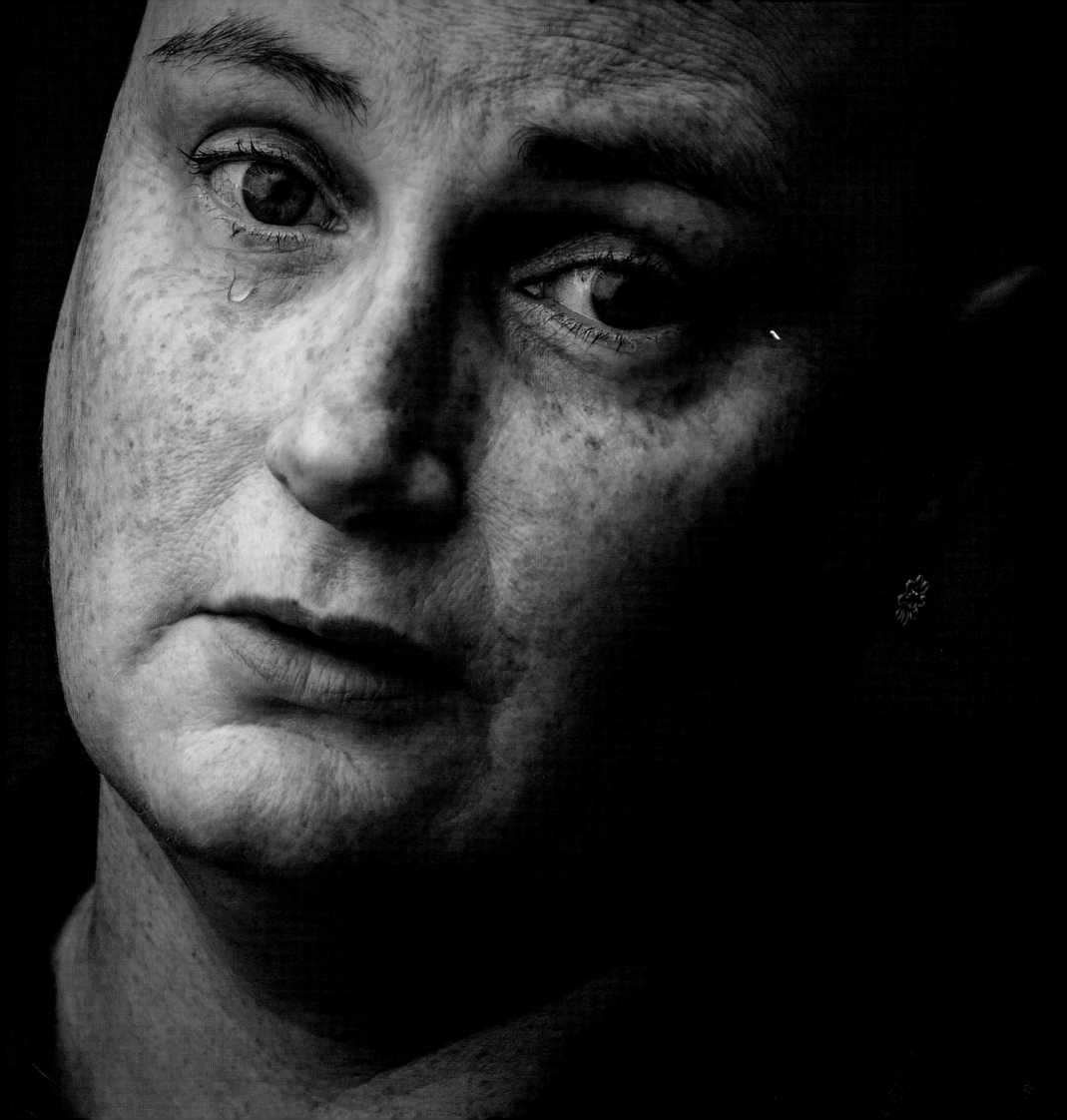

14 DECEMBER 2017

Today, I had to go to the hospital for a prone table stereotactic biopsy, so they could have a better look at the calcification in my breast. This close to Christmas, and with Andy having so much time off over the holiday period, his mum and dad came with me to this appointment instead (my parents live in France).

It started with a normal mammogram, after which I was taken to the procedure room. This has got to be one of the weirdest things I have ever done. I changed into the hospital gown and then had to lie on the table that had a hole in it. My left breast was held out of the way, and the right one was made to hang down through the hole in the table. This hanging breast was then clamped tightly between two plates like those used for mammograms, and the table was raised above the heads of the nurses and radiologists.

I felt like it was a cross between a medieval torture chamber and the cow milking machine, such a strange experience.

I was given a local anaesthetic in the nipple, and a small incision was made in my breast. A needle connected to a vacuum machine across the room was inserted into the tissue and core samples were taken out of the areas of calcification. They had to make sure they had samples that contained the calcification, so the cores were examined there and then.

I watched samples of my breast tissue being walked across the room in a Petrie dish to be examined under a microscope. Once the samples were taken, my breast had to remain clamped between the plates to keep the pressure on the area for about 10 minutes to reduce the bruising. I hate to think what it would look like without the pressure as it has turned into a rainbow of different colours, even having had the pressure applied to the area.

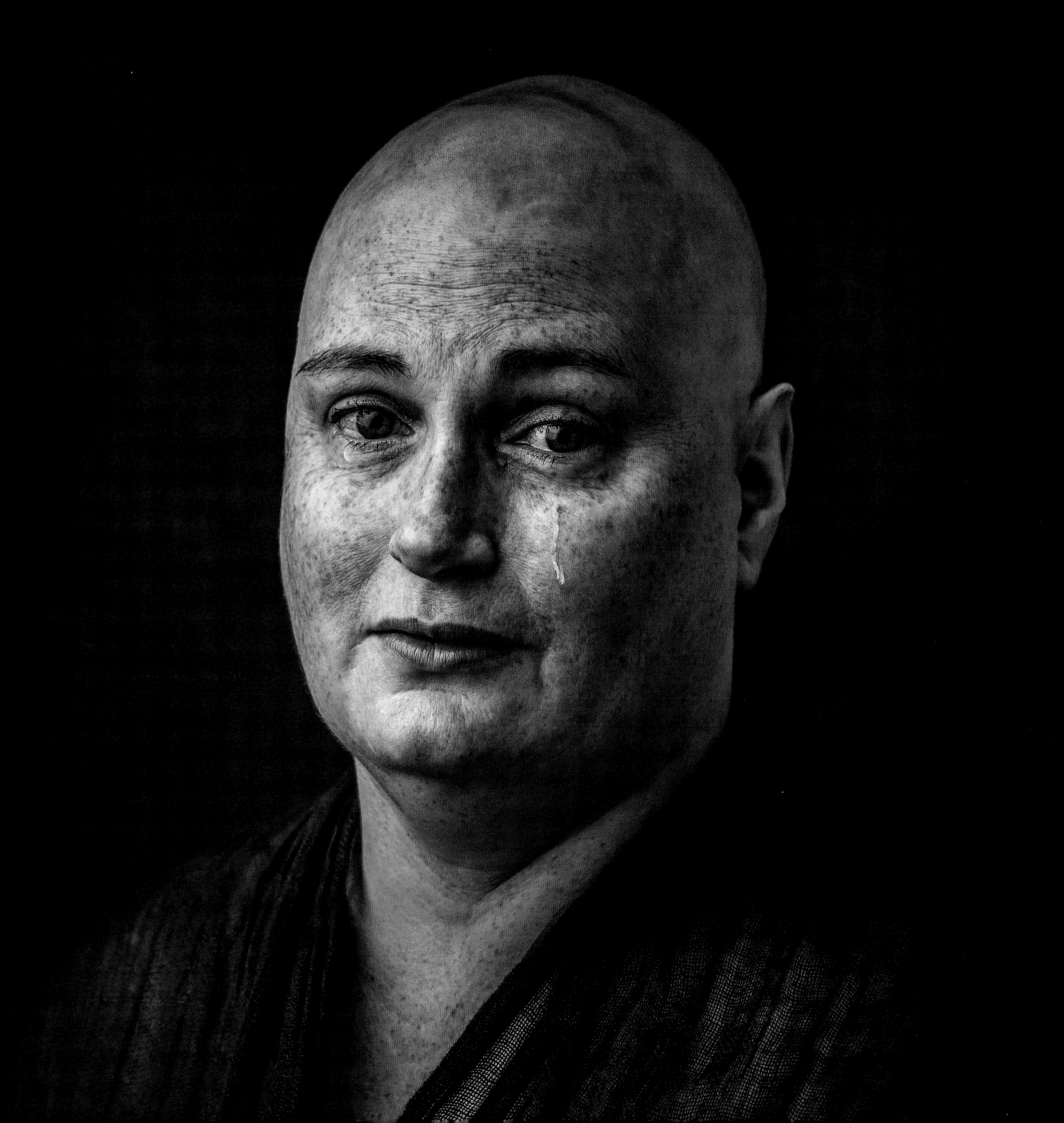

21 DECEMBER 2017

My daughters were off school today, and Andy came home early so we could all go to the hospital. I wanted someone to go with me into the room and both Andy and my older daughter, Hannah, were squeamish and said they'd be sick if they had to watch needles going into me. My younger daughter, Caitlin, went with me instead.

I was having a microbubble test. This is a special test that was pioneered at the Somerfield Hospital in Maidstone, and it involves a solution of microbubbles being injected into the breast to help the path of travel to the lymph nodes be seen with ultrasound. Caitlin held my hand as yet again I had a local anaesthetic injected into my nipple. She watched as a small incision was made and a sample taken with a biopsy needle. The first spring-loaded needle shot into my lymph node, and it felt like someone shoved a spear into my armpit. I yelped, and the radiologist gave me another shot of the local anaesthetic. After that, I didn't have any more pain, and the rest of the samples were taken.

Once I left the room, the practice manager asked me to wait as my breast surgeon would like to have a quick word with me. Andy and I went into the room to see him, and he told me that the results were back and that my cancer was HER2 positive, so we could go ahead and plan surgery as there was no need for genetic testing.

The date of my surgery will be confirmed next week. I then saw the breast care nurse, and she gave me a beautiful patchwork heart-shaped cushion made by volunteers in a group called the "Hearty Quilters." It is to go under my arm following the lymph node biopsy and after my mastectomy, as the area will be very tender. I am very touched by the kindness of strangers donating their time and beautiful cushions.

Now, I need to try and enjoy my Christmas, although I do think Santa could've been a bit nicer to me!

22 DECEMBER 2017

Andy is now off for Christmas, and my friend, Gemma, asked whether I fancied joining her for a coffee. I had just noticed that she blocked me on Facebook, and was wondering what I had done to upset her when she messaged me. It was all very weird, but she asked me to meet her at a nearby coffee shop.

I waited inside for her, and she appeared doing a Facebook live video to a group of local photographers. She had presents and a huge bunch of flowers for me. In the middle of the flowers was a Strelitzia, also known as a "Bird of Paradise". We had them growing in our garden in my childhood home, so they mean a lot to me. It turns out Gemma had unfriended me so that she could block me from seeing her conversations with the other ladies in the group while they arranged a collection to buy me a gift so that I know they are thinking of me at this difficult time.

Gemma had put so much thought into buying the gifts. I got body lotion, hand cream and room fragrance sticks from Rituals. They were all labeled "art of happiness" with lovely sayings on each item. I also received a beautiful bracelet with a paper crane charm on it. The crane represents healing. I was so touched by this kindness from my fellow photographers I just wanted to cry.

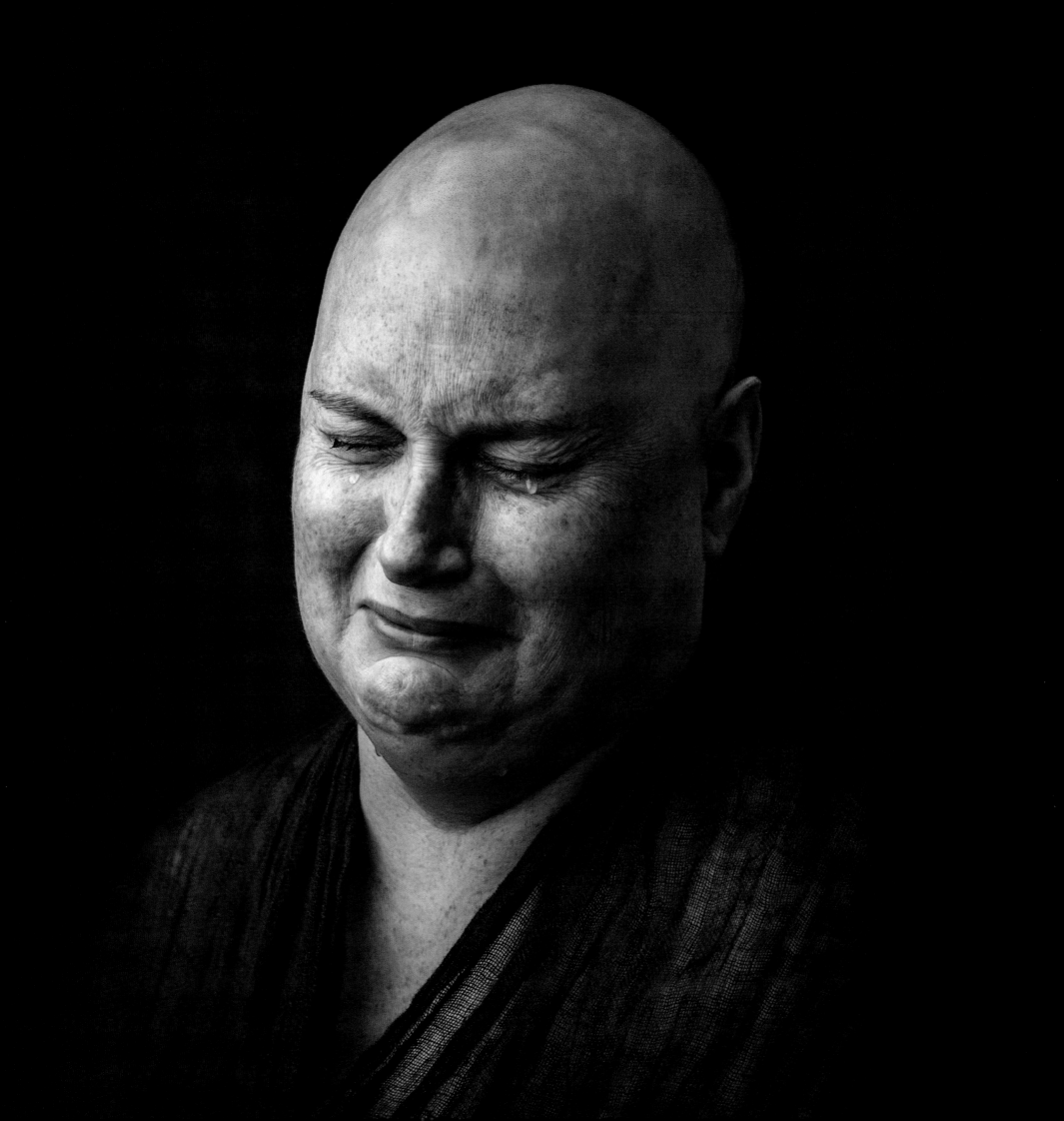

25 DECEMBER 2017

Christmas went by in a haze and really was a non-event this year. Luckily the girls are teenagers, so it didn't bother them too much. We did go to Andy's parents for Christmas dinner and had a nice relaxing day.

28 DECEMBER 2017

Another appointment today, and we arrived at outpatients. The car park was completely deserted, and we couldn't get in through the door to the outpatients' department. Eventually, we got to the main entrance of the hospital and found out where the clinic was. It turns out that the floor was being replaced in outpatients, so we needed to go a different way to get there.

I didn't find out much more than we already knew, other than my surgery will be on 8 January, and will be followed by chemotherapy and Herceptin, which is a targeted therapy and the new wonder drug. I will come home with a drain (a catheter from my wound into a plastic bag to collect fluid) after surgery, so I was given some cotton bags in which to carry them around. The nurse showed me a "softie," which is a post-surgery bra insert. She took her time to talk to me about the mastectomy procedure.

One of the main things I am worried about with everything coming is losing my hair if I have to have chemotherapy, and I asked if that would happen. I was told it's more than likely. It's funny how in the face of things, us women are so worried about something like losing our hair.

29 DECEMBER 2017

With potential baldness looming, I decided to take control and get my long hair cut into a short style. This is something I would never have been brave enough to do if I didn't have cancer, but I want to donate my hair to the Little Princess Trust, a charity that makes wigs for little girls who have hair loss due to cancer treatment or some other illness.

We went as a family for a walk-in appointment at a new salon. I was very nervous, and we had to wait for ages, and when it was finally my turn, Caitlin (my younger daughter) videoed it. I kept telling myself it's only hair and it will grow back. The radio happened to be on, and I could hear Coldplay singing "Fix You" in the background while my hair was cut. It seemed very appropriate. I put my hair into a plastic bag, ready to post to the Little Princess Trust.

31 DECEMBER 2017

New Year's Eve.

This was the first time I had seen my friends since my new haircut, and I was very self-conscious going out. It was just a few of us going around to another friend's house, and we had a good evening playing Ping-Pong, Prosecco, and chatting.

Midnight was very emotional to both Andy and me, as the realisation hit us that we were now in the year when all my treatments will happen. There were more than a few tears from both of us. However, I felt very loved and cared for by Andy, which is a blessing.

2 JANUARY 2018

I have really been struggling to sleep. So much is going around my head about my operation and treatment.

I posted in a Breast Cancer support group on Facebook asking for tips on sleeping. A few people mentioned Twilight Spray and Sleepy Cream from Lush, so I decided to go into town and have a look.

In the store, I picked up the last bottle of Twilight Spray. It was hard smelling it with all the fragrances from the soaps. I wandered over to look for the Sleepy Cream, and also spotted a Dream Cream. A staff member came over to me to ask if I wanted some help, and I explained where I had heard about this cream and spray, and I also explained that I would have quite a sensitive skin during chemotherapy.

In the end, I decided to leave the cream and start the Twilight body spray to help me sleep. I followed him to the till where he told me that they were allowed to do a random act of kindness each day, and that he wanted me to have the spray at no cost. I nearly cried at this generosity. It was a £20 bottle, which was given as a gift by a complete stranger. How amazing is that! And it smells lovely!

3 JANUARY 2018

Today was my pre-operation assessment appointment. I haven't got much to say about this. It was just lots of tests: blood, EKG, weight, height, MRSA swab and lots of forms to sign!

As I am classed as obese, I have extra risks during surgery, but the one that freaked me out was I could stay awake. That really is the stuff of nightmares! And when they mentioned a urine test, I said, "No, I cannot possibly be pregnant, as I have no womb!" I had a hysterectomy several years ago, so that would be more than a miracle.

4 JANUARY 2018

I can finally say it out loud, "I HAVE CANCER!"

I can say it, but the words still feel strange. I feel as though I am living in somebody else's body. It is so surreal!

As a photographer, I am very fortunate to have many talented friends, and my close friend, Claire, came all the way from Durham to Kent to see me. I don't really like being in front of the camera, but I didn't want to regret not having photographs taken before surgery changed my appearance. Claire used my studio and my camera to do a photo shoot of me, showing off "my assets." I'm not one to show off my body, as I have gained so much weight over the years, so being photographed in minimal clothing was not something I would have been comfortable doing, but Claire was great and put me at ease, and we had a lot of fun. It really gave me the opportunity to experience what it is like on the other side of the camera, which has helped me grow as a photographer too. There were a few tears along the way as we spoke of what was scheduled in the forthcoming year, but it was a wonderful, positive experience, and I'm very glad that I did it.

(Reading back over this, almost six months later, I am still very glad I had my photos taken. I edited the images, but I hadn't looked at them since my surgery. In one of the photos, I left the bruise from a biopsy, as I felt that it was part of my story.) I love the photos, and I'm so grateful to Claire for taking them for me.

Claire has given me a "Little Miss Naughty" mug to remind me to keep my "naughty" side, and a little cuddly elephant toy. We were doing some crafting, and I attached a pink ribbon for breast cancer to the elephant's ear. I also have a cuddly rhino toy, as I love rhinos and regularly visit them at Howletts Wildlife Park. I also attached a couple of breast cancer motifs to the rhino, and I named her Hope. Claire thought Faith was a good name for the little elephant, and I decided to create an Instagram account for them, to document my journey, using them as mascots.

Claire stayed until Sunday morning and then headed home. I was sad to see her go but look forward to seeing her soon at the Guild of Photographers awards next month.

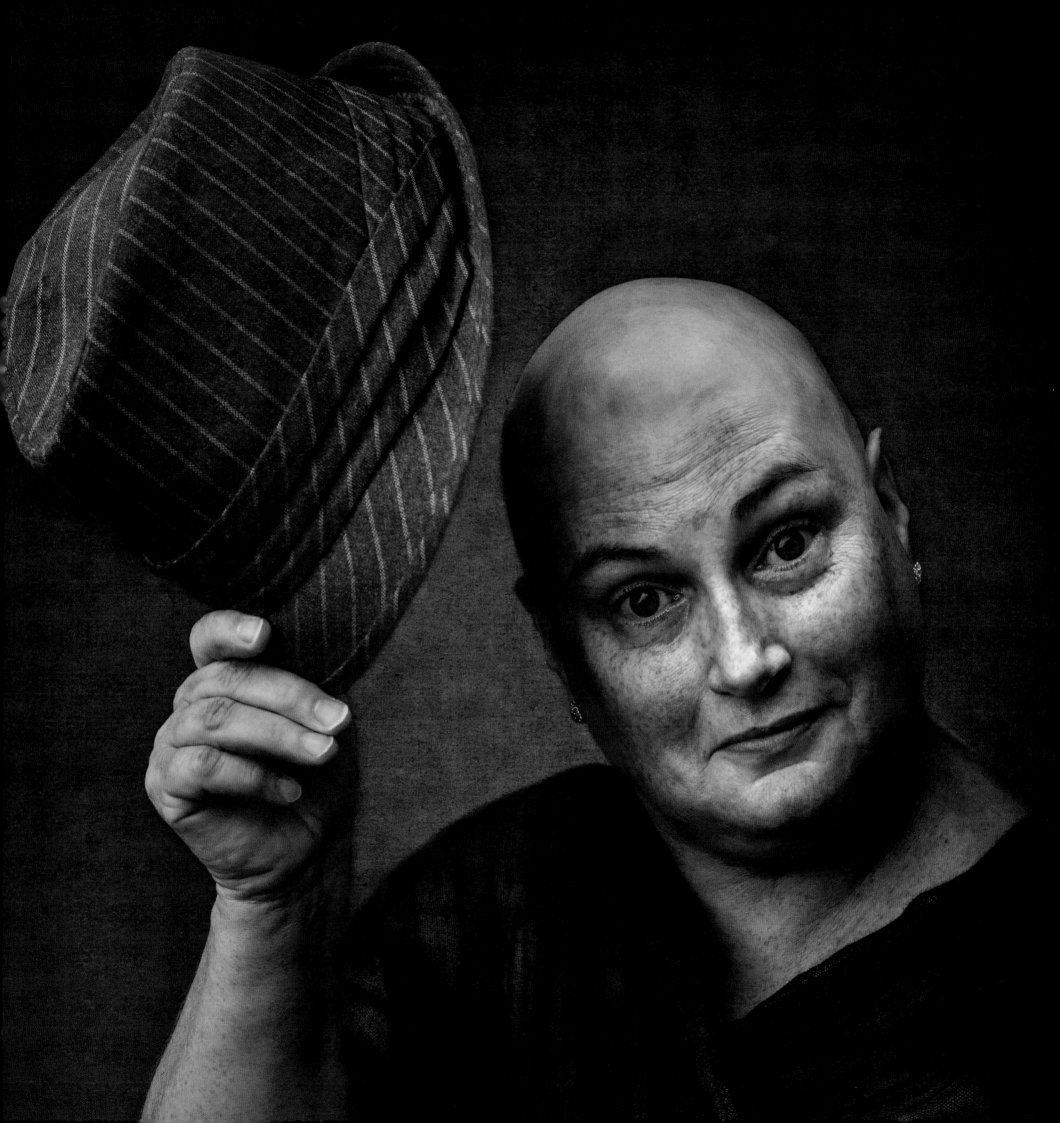

Operation Day!

I was nil by mouth from 6:30 a.m., so I had a quick slice of toast and a cup of coffee while the girls got ready for school.

We had to be at the hospital to be admitted at 9 a.m. On the way, I got something in my eye and scratched it, so I arrived with a red, swollen and watery eye, looking like I had been crying for a week.

The porter took us to my room, and once I changed into my hospital gown and delightful surgical stockings, I had to go down to nuclear medicine to be injected with a radioactive isotope.

We sat in outpatients waiting to be seen, and then we were taken through to a room with a big machine and a photograph of trees on the ceiling above where I lay. Andy held my hand, and my breast was injected for the final time while conscious. For a brief moment, I want to shout out "STOP" and object, won't a radioactive isotope give me cancer? Doh!

The isotope and a blue dye are used to help locate the sentinel or guard nodes, which are the first nodes to which a tumour drains. They are later analysed in the laboratory, as a needle biopsy can miss cancer cells from time to time.

I then had the scan before going back to my room.

Time went by really slowly, and it seemed like ages before we were finally seen by the anaesthetist and breast surgeon. A nurse then accompanied me as we walked down to the theatre. Andy followed as far as the theatre doors and then hugged me. I was a bit emotional at this point, but I reconciled myself, as I wasn't saying goodbye to my breast – I was saying F-off, cancer!

In the pre-theatre area, I met the team there for my operation. They asked me to lie down on the bed, but it felt a bit high, so they get a step for me, as I am rather short at 5ft 1.

A cannula was inserted, and I was shown some dressings as an alternative to Tegaderm, which causes my skin to blister. We decided on the thicker, padded dressing which is usually for joints. I told my anaesthetist about my fear, after my pre-op assessment, about being awake during surgery, and he reassured me it was very unlikely. I felt the ache as he injected the anaesthetic into my cannula, and I vaguely remember something about a joke and counting down from 100 but I was too sleepy by then and my eyelids were getting heavy….

I heard someone say my name and briefly opened my eyes. I was aware of a nurse sitting near to me talking, and I could hear the beeping of machines and the faint whoosh of oxygen coming through the mask I had covering my nose and mouth. She asked if I was in any pain, then I pointed to the centre of my chest and under my arm.

The rest of the day felt like something from a movie as I drifted in and out of consciousness. I can't recall the trip back from recovery to the ward, but I do remember getting a brief glimpse of Andy and my daughters as I was wheeled into my room.

Caitlin was in the chair next to my bed. She reached out to take my hand....

I came back from the theatre looking like a smurf with a blue face from the dye they used. It was a bit of a shock for my kids to see me like this. Hannah fainted the moment she saw me and had to be taken out of the room.

Andy took the girls home, and the rest of the night consisted of waking up each time my blood pressure and temperature was taken and from the noise of the air pillows inflating and deflating round my calves to keep the blood flow and prevent thrombosis.

9 JANUARY 2018

A nurse brought me a cup of tea and biscuit at about 5:30 a.m., as I didn't have my sandwich last night. I was too sleepy and didn't feel well enough.

I was helped to have a wash, and I changed into my pyjamas and sat in the chair for breakfast. I ordered it before my operation, and it seemed like a good idea at the time. I was now presented with a full English breakfast, a honey and banana smoothie, and a cup of coffee. It looked very tasty, but I didn't want to eat at all.

Andy came back in after the consultant had seen me. I can't remember much about what he said to me in the post-anaesthetic fog, but I did ask him how much my breast weighed, as Andy, Claire and my kids were taking bets on how much it would be. I can't remember exactly what it weighed, but it was roughly 1.5 kg, I think. Wow, that's heavy! I could be slimmer of the week at my weight loss club with that amount coming off.

I spent a lot of time sleeping.

I had fishcakes with lemon mayonnaise for lunch and salmon for supper (bit of a fishy day), and fresh fruit salad is my favourite for pudding, as I didn't want anything too rich.

Andy's parents visited just after lunch and Andy came in a bit later. My sister-in-law visited at about 5:30 p.m. and brought me a lovely soft grey blanket, so I can snuggle on the sofa and keep warm once I'm home. Her husband, Andy's brother, arrived a while later with my nieces. It was lovely to see them. I also had some friends visit a bit later, and they gave me some lovely headscarves for when I lose my hair.

10 JANUARY 2018

I had a cinnamon swirl and toast for breakfast. Another friend, Lydia, who has also had breast cancer, came to visit, and we chatted about her recent wedding and her experience with cancer. It was good to chat with someone who has travelled a similar journey. She helped me to get dressed and packed my things for me, and after a pesto chicken sandwich for lunch with the obligatory fruit salad, Andy came to fetch me, and I was allowed to go home.

I had to wait for the porter with the wheelchair to take me to the car. I felt strangely emotional as I was wheeled out of the ward and past the reception desk. I have no idea why, but I cried.

Home sweet home!

I came home and went straight to bed. I have a drain from my wound, which has to be emptied and measured every 24 hours. It can be removed once the fluid measures less than 50 ml in 24 hours, and at the moment, it is just over 100 ml.

Another friend came to visit. Her son was diagnosed with stage 4 lymphoma last year, and his last chemo was before Christmas. He has sent me some lovely messages via Facebook, offering support, which is so sweet and thoughtful, as he is only 17 years old.

Stephanie, another friend who is also a photographer, came to visit, and she brought me a beautiful bunch of flowers. I am really looking forward to going to the Guild awards with her in a few weeks, as she is driving me up there and we are sharing a room. Bring on the road trip!

14 JANUARY 2018

Andy has to go back to work tomorrow, so my mother is arriving to look after me for a few days. It is nice to know that she will be here, so I won't be alone when Andy goes back to work.

My dressings got wet, so we had to change them. I was surprised by the large size of the cut!

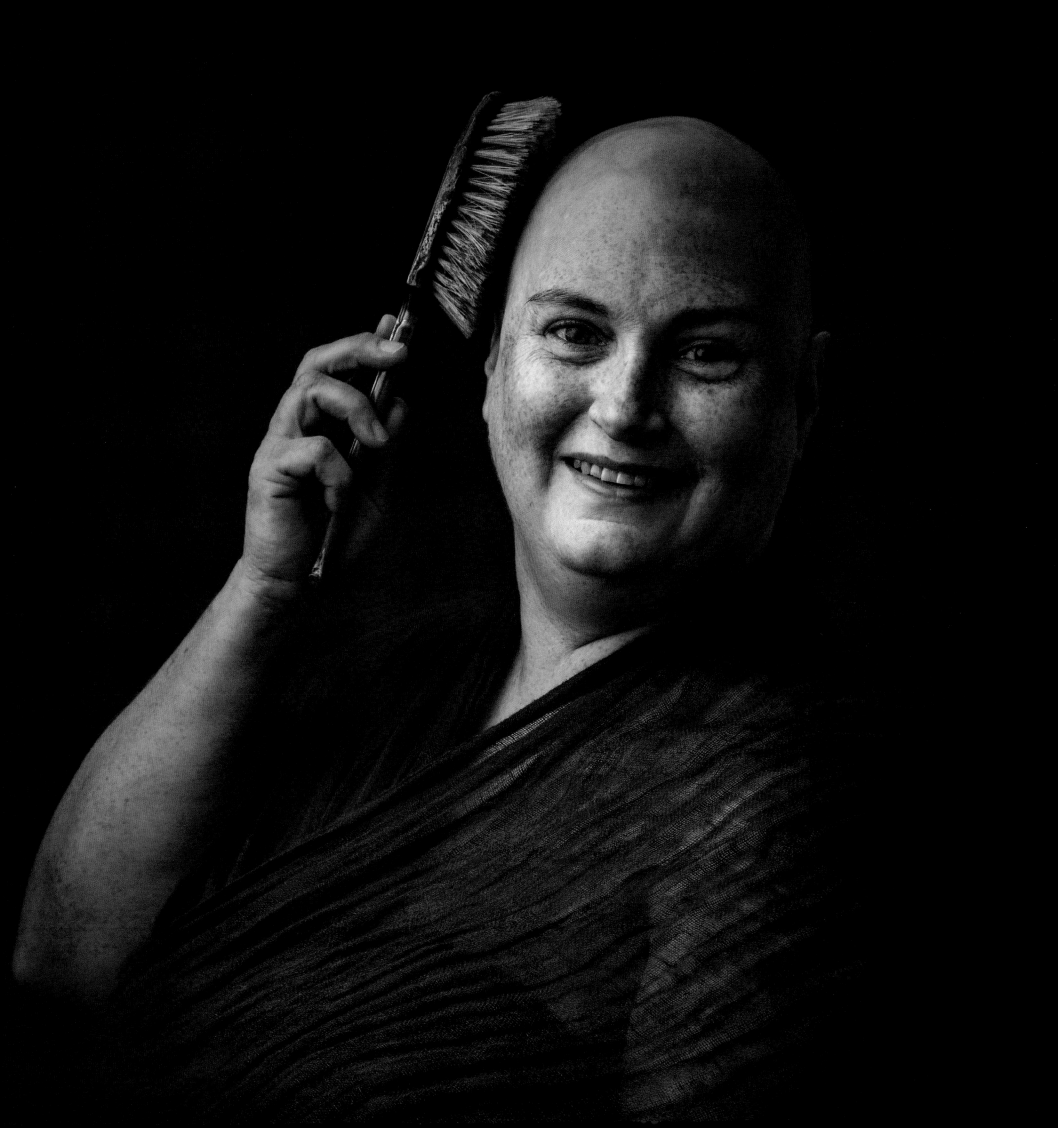

I have to go back to see my consultant this evening, and hopefully, my dressings will come off. Although I have a suspicion that the drain will have to stay in a while longer, I pray that I am wrong.

I was just chuckling to myself, as we have realised that Andy was giving me the wrong dose of Oramorph! I was supposed to have 5ml/10g, but he was giving me 10 ml, double the dose I should've been taking! No wonder I was almost pain-free and high as a kite!

I haven't been sleeping very well, and I am pacing at night with twitchy legs. It is very annoying! My pain isn't as bad as I thought, and most of it is under my arm. I am trying to do my physiotherapy exercises regularly to keep the area mobile, but it is still very difficult.

I had some phantom pains in the nipple that is no longer there, but the weirdest feeling is when I drink something. It feels like the liquid is spilling out of my oesophagus and trickling down the inside of my chest. It feels awful and uncomfortable with drinks from the fridge, but warm drinks don't hurt as much. I asked about it in a breast cancer group on Facebook, and lots of people have experienced it. It seems it goes away eventually, but one lady said it lasted seven years! Yikes!

I had a bit of a meltdown on Sunday evening. Everyone was posting about what a great time they had at the photography convention, and it suddenly struck me how messed up my year is going to be. I had planned on entering into the Guild of Photographers Monthly Competition every month, but I won't be able to be near kids or babies during chemotherapy. I planned on submitting my master craftsman panel, and now, that has to wait. I am scared of losing my creativity and passion for photography, and also really worried about keeping my business afloat!

Well, that appointment did not go to plan!

In the car on the way to the hospital, Andy and I discussed the worst-case scenario, which was more surgery if the cancer had spread to my lymph nodes. We arrived and were taken by the breast care nurse to the treatment room to have my dressings removed. The wound was fine, but I felt a bit sick when the area was cleaned. After that, my drain was removed. Yay! Wow, it hurt! I felt like the tube was almost at my shoulders and I actually screamed as it came out. The nurse did comment that it seemed to go in a long way. The area was re-dressed, and we went through to see the consultant.

I was told that the tumour was removed along with the 110mm section of DCIS. My breast surgeon then went on to discuss the lymph node biopsy and told me that they had found cancer cells in both lymph nodes that were removed. That means that I have to have another surgery to remove my remaining lymph nodes in what is known as an axillary node clearance. It is a similar surgery to my mastectomy, but the cut under my arm will be extended to allow access to the rest of the nodes, of which there could be up to 24, and they will be removed. I will need another drain!

So, it turns out that my tumour was Grade 3 and my cancer, stage 3, not stage 2 as we previously thought. We've been told to expect at least 6 to 8 months of living around breast cancer. Surgery is now booked, and I will only have a few days to recover if I am allowed to go to the photography awards as planned. Last year, I was the winner of the contemporary portraiture image of the year, and I don't imagine winning anything two years in a row, although that would be nice, but it is such a fun weekend with like-minded people!

I was very emotional and tearful; as I really don't want to miss the awards, as that is the only thing I have to look forward to this year. I have to go to a different hospital further away from home so that I can have my next operation before the Guild of Photography Awards, but I chose to do that to get the surgery out of the way sooner, rather than wait a few extra days. I want more time to recover before I go away, so every day counts!

Andy was very upset by this latest development, and there were tears on the way home when I announced that "I am not going to die"! I dreaded telling my mother when we got home but it turned out she already thought I was stage 3 and wasn't shocked by the news. Hannah was very upset, as after the fainting episodes last time, she won't be allowed back into the hospital when I have the next surgery, so she knows she won't be able to visit me this time.

18 JANUARY 2018

I had a lovely surprise today when the postman arrived. He delivered a lovely bunch of flowers from the Guild of Photographers. It put a big smile on my face and really cheered me up knowing how caring and supportive all my photography friends are!

Take two getting rid of this bloody cancer!

I was a bit upset that Caitlin didn't even bother to give me a hug or wish me luck when she went out the door this morning to catch the bus. Hannah was being very caring towards me, which was nice.

I had to be at the hospital by 12 noon, and I've been nil by mouth since 7 a.m. In order to take my mind off things, we went and wandered around the shops in town, and we grabbed a coffee. Well, Andy had a coffee, and I got a bottle of water, which was the only thing allowed until 10 a.m., after which time, even clear liquids had to stop. We bought some therapeutic colouring books and felt tip pens to keep me occupied during all the waiting.

We finally arrived at the hospital, and I was checked into my room, which has a garden view. The nurses were all very friendly. My breast surgeon popped in and got me to sign the consent form, and a while later, the anaesthetist came and went through the usual checks.

I then got changed into my hospital gown and had to get into bed, as you go down to theatre on your bed here, rather than walking. I had to leave Andy at the ward, and off I went. I chatted with the anaesthetist while he prepared me for surgery. For the first time ever, they struggled to find a vein, so it took quite a lot of squeezing and pushing on my arm to make veins appear. Eventually, they managed to insert a cannula into a vein in my forearm and anaesthetic was injected while we discussed having a Portacath inserted for chemotherapy instead of going through this each time! I felt myself getting woozy …

I woke up in recovery with a man talking to me, and I realised it was my nurse. I could see a clock on the wall and the time changed by at least five minutes every time I opened my eyes. The nurse put an oxygen mask on my face to help me wake up, and after about half an hour, I was taken back to my room.

Andy was waiting for me, but I was too sleepy to really talk to him. A bit later, he headed off so I could get some sleep, and my night of blood pressure, temperature and oxygen started as well as the regular click, brrrrr, pffew of the cuffs around my feet as they inflated and deflated to keep the blood circulating through my legs. The cuffs mean that I couldn't get out of bed during the night and the poor nurse had to bring me a bedpan three times. They are horrible things and make you feel like you're sitting in your own urine — well, I guess you are! I was paranoid about stinking of wee by the morning!

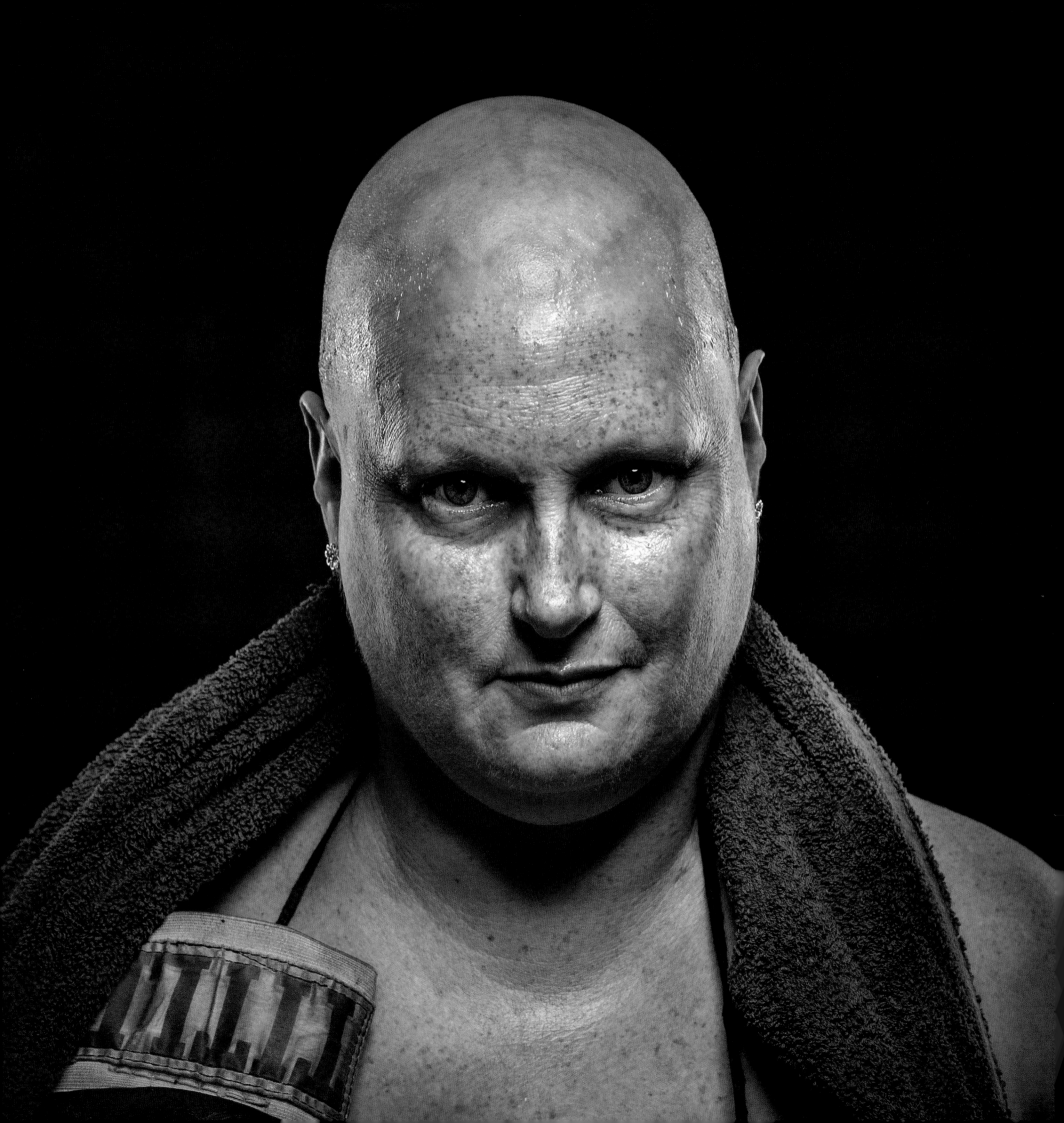

23 JANUARY 2018

It was a bit of a sleepless night with the foot cuffs and blood pressure checks. I finally felt hungry about 4 a.m. and had a cup of tea and a Jammie Dodger, one of my favourite biscuits.

One of the perks of being in hospital — 4 a.m. Jammie Dodgers!

The nurses helped me get a shower and wash this morning, so I felt much better after that. Andy arrived in the late morning. I had broccoli and stilton soup, risotto balls and crème brûlée for lunch. This afternoon, my friend Jane came to see me, and it was great to catch up.

Everyone has left now, and I have just finished a delicious steak dinner. I was very impressed, and it was nicer than many restaurants in which I have eaten.

I managed to look at my new cut, and there was a lot of extra flesh missing, and I am concave under my arm. I look like a shark has bitten me! I spoke to one of the nurses about it, and she said that they take away a lot of tissue and the lymph nodes get separated in the laboratory.

I am quite sore tonight, and I just found what I thought was a hair sticking out of my mastectomy scar. I pulled it, and it appeared out of my cut. I think it was one of the internal stitches peeping out. A nurse has now put a dressing over the stitch and it should eventually drop off. They said I can go home tomorrow.

28 JANUARY 2018

I have been home for a few days now, and my drain is really bothering me. I messaged my breast care nurse, and she is going to have a look for me tomorrow to see if it can be removed. It was still producing a lot of fluid on Friday (over 200 ml), but it has really slowed over the last two days, so I am hoping it comes out.

29 JANUARY 2018

Yes, the drain is out! The point of entry was starting to feel like it had acid on it and was burning every time I jolted it or moved around. This time, I took Co-Codamol before it was removed, and it wasn't nearly as painful. It also helped that the drain didn't go in as far as the previous one had. I now just have a small strip of surgical tape over the cut (the type the plastic surgeons use to minimise scarring).

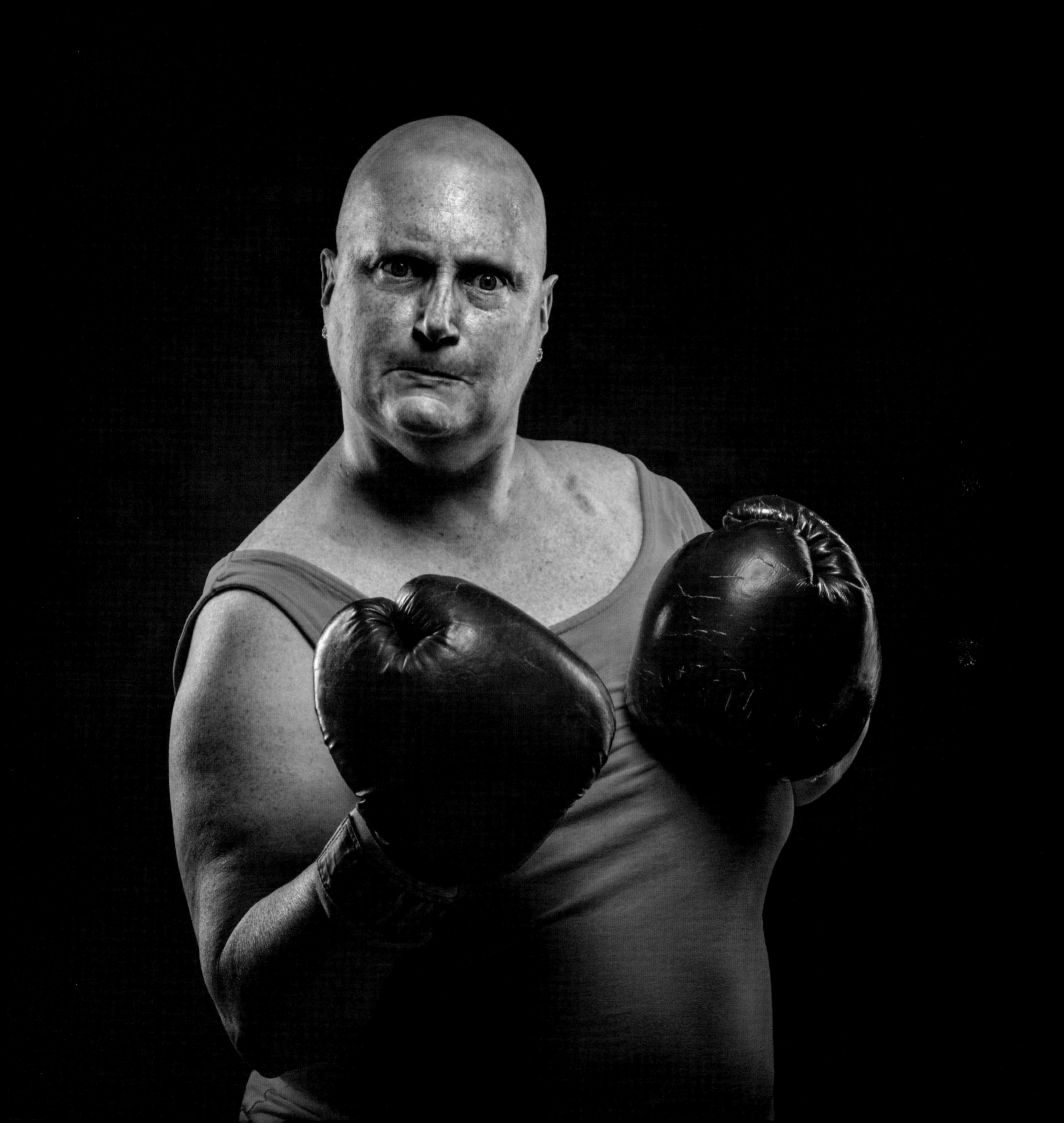

30 JANUARY 2018

I had my follow-up appointment after my axillary node clearance today. I've had a further 18 lymph nodes removed, and only one of them showed signs of cancer, so thankfully, that should be the end of surgery for now. I can be passed on to the oncology department.

I am really excited as I can go to the Guild of Photographers' awards weekend.   Yippee!

1 FEBRUARY 2018

Yay! Girly road trip.

My friend Stephanie picked me up, and we drove to meet another friend at a hotel where we are staying overnight, so we can get an early start tomorrow. We met up with some other photographers at the pub for a meal. It was a lovely evening, but I started to ache and feel under the weather. We didn't linger after dinner and went back to the hotel, and I was very grateful to be able to get my clothes away from my wound. The skin is very sensitive and a bit red and swollen. We had a fun night, in spite of it!

2 FEBRUARY 2018

We rose bright and early and headed off for a day of photography training. The redness in my chest has gone down a bit. It is so great to see so many friends, and the support they have shown me is amazing. Stephanie has been really fantastic, and she made sure I had a little rest at lunchtime, so I didn't get too tired.

We had cocktails in the bar before dinner, and I got to catch up with a lot more friends. We had a large table booked for dinner, and the food was much better than I remember it being in previous years. After dinner, we went back to the bar, although I was then on soft drinks, I was soon very tired, and at 10 pm I had to go back to the room.

The windows were wide open to let in some fresh air, and it is absolutely freezing! It took me forever to warm up, and when Stephanie got back to the room, we realised that the other window was still open. No wonder it was so cold. In spite of the cold, I woke up sweating, and surprised there was no human-shaped sweat mark on the bedclothes!

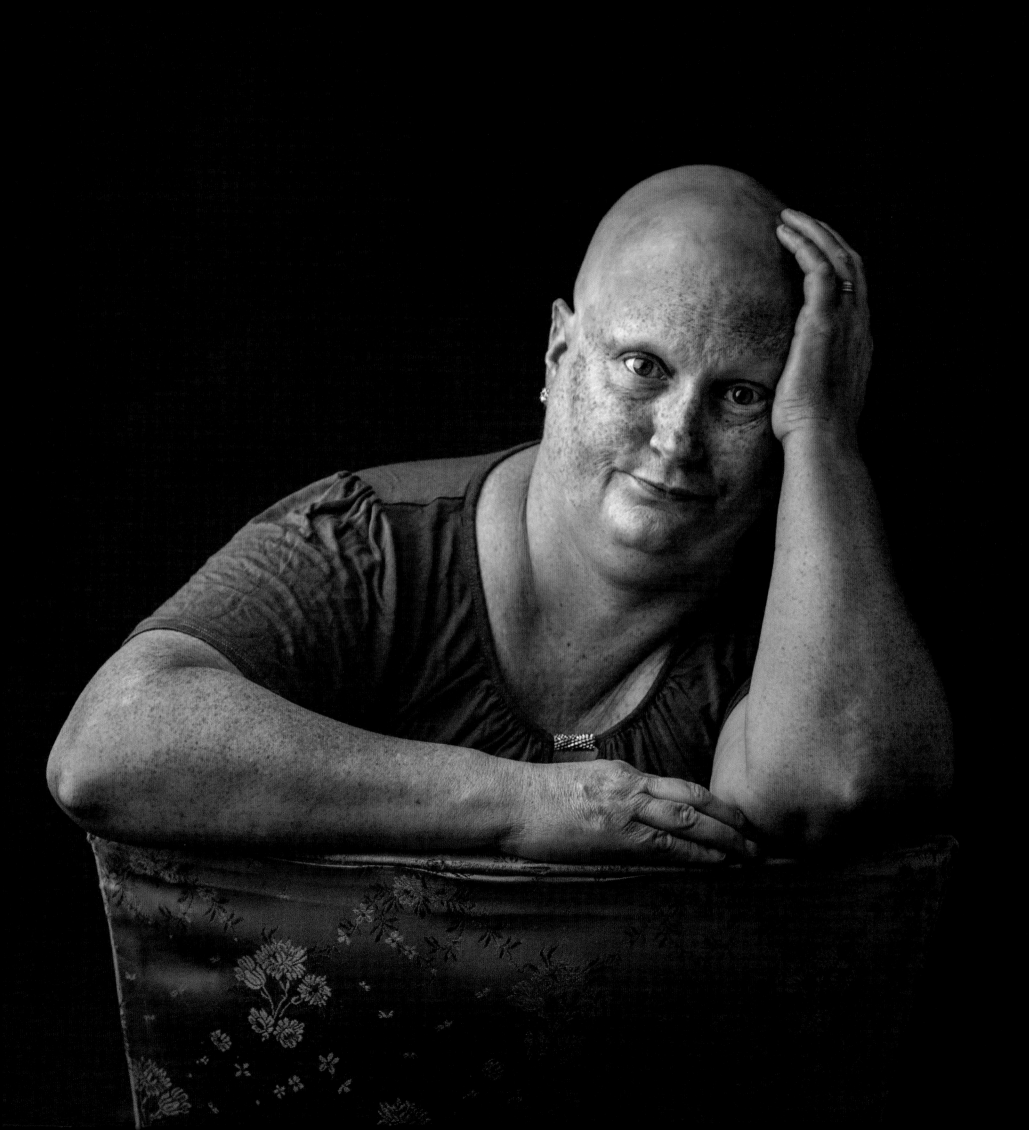

3 FEBRUARY 2018

My chest was a bit redder this morning, but I carried on with my day. I showed a friend a bit later, and she agreed that it looked redder and more swollen than last night. Another friend, who is a GP, said it looked infected and told me to ring the NHS out-of-hours service, as I needed antibiotics.

It took ages to get through, but when I did, the lady was very helpful. She asked if I had a temperature, but I didn't know as I have just come off Hormone Replacement Therapy, which I have been taking since my hysterectomy. I didn't know if these sweats were from this or from having a temperature. After going through everything, I was given an appointment at 3 p.m. at the local hospital with the out-of-hours GP. Stephanie took me, and came in with me, to see the GP.

The doctor had a look and wanted to admit me to a ward for IV antibiotics and fluids. We explained that we were only there for one more night for the photography awards and that we were heading back to Kent tomorrow. She agreed to give me oral antibiotics, and yes, you guessed it, I couldn't drink alcohol.

I was told to go straight back to the hospital if it got worse and to contact the breast clinic on Monday to get it looked at. Stephanie decided not to drink alcohol that night, just in case something went wrong and we had to go back to the hospital. I said it wasn't necessary, but she insisted. We got back to the hotel and got dressed for the awards. I couldn't face anything against my chest, so there was no chance of a bra or a softie, and I had to go to the awards with just one boob! At least, I was with understanding friends, so wasn't too embarrassed.

It was a fantastic night at the awards, and I was very overwhelmed to be awarded the 2017 special recognition award. I was quite tired, so we headed to bed much earlier than I usually would on an awards night. It was an amazing night, though, and I loved seeing everybody.

4 FEBRUARY 2018

Time to face reality and head home!

I felt really sad saying goodbye to everyone. There were plenty of hugs and tears and then a long drive home. I felt very tired in the car and was quite relieved to get home. I called the hospital as soon as I got in and explained what had been going on, and I was told to go straight to the ward to be seen. I hadn't even unpacked when we headed to the hospital where the doctor looked at me and drew a line in pen around the red area as a reference. They took a swab and dressed the wound and told me to get an appointment with my consultant, first thing in the morning. We headed home, and I was sound asleep by 8 p.m.

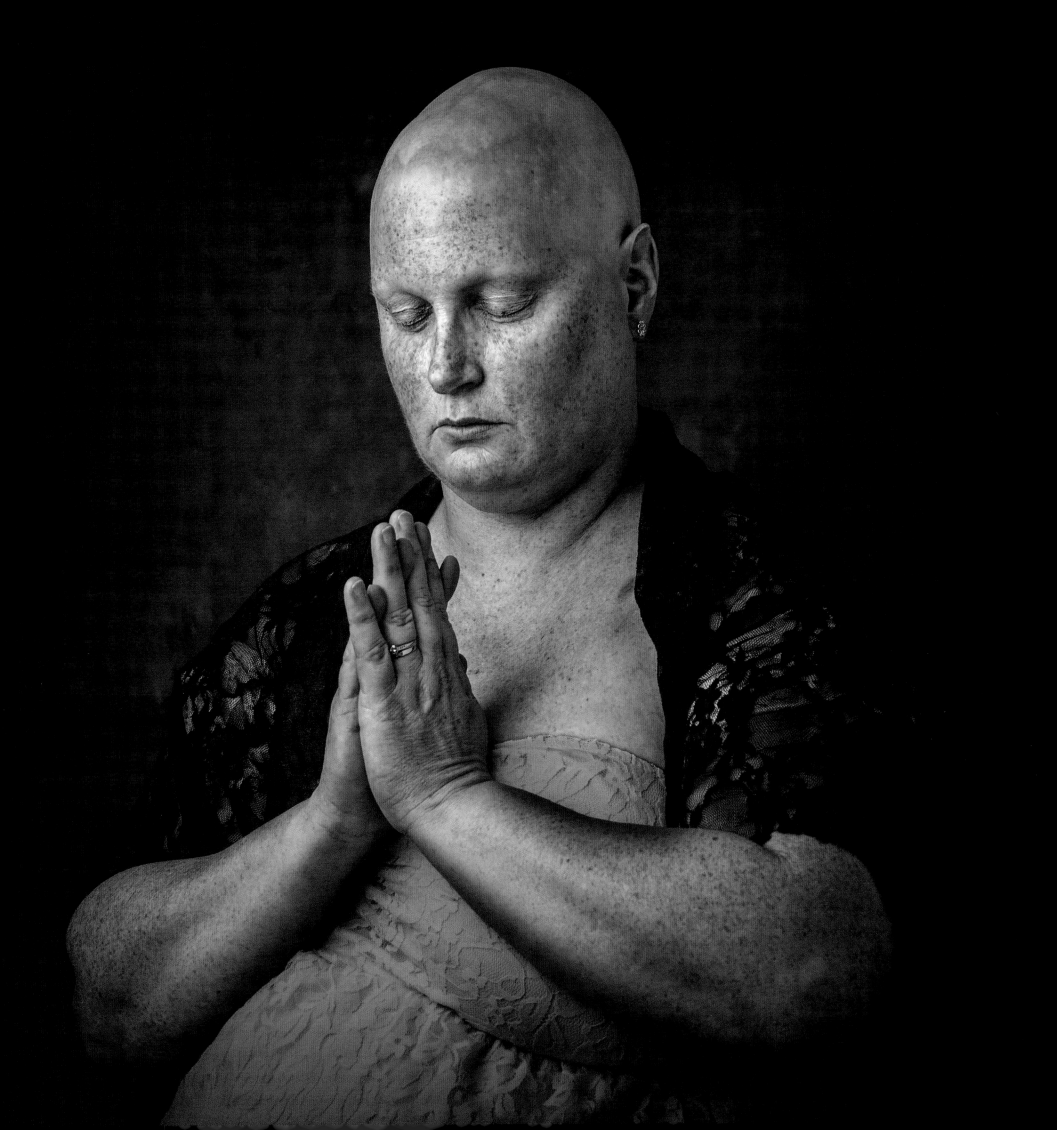

5 FEBRUARY 2018

Andy's parents took me to my appointment with the consultant. He took a look and thought it was probably just a fluid build-up that needed to be drained, so he got a nurse to help him.

It was rather a large needle with a three-way valve on the syringe and some tubing. Thankfully, due to (as my consultant puts it) a rather large knife having cut through my nerves, I didn't feel anything. He started to drain the fluid and had a rather surprised look on his face when it turned out to be pus and not fluid after all. After quite a length of time and several syringes emptied into the dish, he successfully drained 350 ml of pus from my wound. Yuck! A pot of it was sent to the laboratory, and some blood was drawn.

I wasn't allowed to leave the hospital until we had the results, so my breast surgeon went back to the theatre while we waited for the results in the waiting room. They came through a while later, and my CRP levels (the blood test marker for inflammation) after two days of strong antibiotics were at 271 (the normal range is less than 10) and I needed to be admitted immediately. I started off in a bed in special care on the ward as all the other beds were occupied.

My in-laws left me to settle in, and I facetimed my daughter and got her to pack a bag for me, as I wasn't expecting to stay. The consultant came back to see me and said that I would be moved into a proper room soon, as one of his patients was going home shortly. Andy came to see me as soon as he was off work, and I was moved to room 209.

8 FEBRUARY 2018

I was supposed to have an oncology appointment today, but I am still in the hospital with the infection, so my breast surgeon called my oncologist to explain why I couldn't make it. I then received a phone call from the oncologist, and he offered to come and see me in this hospital, rather than me having to make another appointment at the clinic.

He came to see me, and we discussed the plan for treatment. I will be on an ECP protocol and Herceptin, which will be followed by radiotherapy to the chest wall. I need Zoledronic Acid to keep my bone density up, as this is a worry now that I have stopped my HRT. The ZA should also prevent cancer from spreading to my bones. Although my cancer is not oestrogen receptive, my doctors feel it safer for me to stop the HRT, just in case there are a few cells that might be affected by my oestrogen levels.

I also need to arrange a dental checkup before I start chemotherapy, as I can't have dental work done within six weeks of each Zoledronic Acid infusion. I need to have regular cardiology tests as Herceptin can weaken the heart. I will need to have a Portacath fitted to avoid having a cannula every time I have chemotherapy. My oncologist stated it might be worth having my baseline cardiology done and the Portacath fitted while still in the hospital, although there is a chance my infection might prevent this.

So now we know my treatment regime, it will be as follows:

» Epirubicin and Cyclophosphamide every 21 days for 4 cycles.
» Paclitaxel every 14 days for the following 4 cycles
» Herceptin injections every 21 days for 18 cycles
» Zoledronic acid infusions every 6 weeks for 3 cycles along with chemotherapy, and then every 6 months for 3 years, Radiotherapy

I will most likely lose my hair, and I was given the details of a lady who sells wigs. I'll see my oncologist again next week with Andy.

There was the talk of needing more surgery to clean my wound, but it is now looking like I might have a drain fitted instead, so I could be discharged on Saturday.

My breast surgeon said that the Portacath cannot be fitted until the infection has cleared, as it is usually fitted on the right and goes into a vein leading to the heart, so while there is an infection, they can't risk it.

10 FEBRUARY 2018

I was discharged and could go home. I had a hefty dose of our antibiotics — double what is usually prescribed and over two weeks. Now, I need to rest and call if I have any problems or if my wound needs draining again. I managed to avoid going home without a drain, and I am so relieved. I have a follow-up appointment in the next couple of weeks, and then I'll be passed onto oncology and be able to get on with chemotherapy.

15 FEBRUARY 2018

Busy day!

I am booked in for my Portacath to be inserted tomorrow, but it may be postponed if my infection hasn't cleared enough. I had to have another MRSA swab as it's been more than four weeks since the last one. The nurse thinks that they might insert my Portacath on the left to allow for radiotherapy on my right-hand side.

Andy has taken the day off to take me to my appointments.

First stop was the dentist, as I needed a full check prior to going on Zoledronic acid which can cause osteonecrosis of the jaw. I won't be able to have any dental treatment for six weeks after each infusion, which basically rules out any dental work for 6 months. The dentist did a really thorough checkup with several x-rays. She picked up slight lip between one tooth and a filling which may attract food, so this needed to be filed smooth. Another filling showed some lighter areas which may be early decay, so she prescribed some double fluoride toothpaste, and I have to have another appointment to refill a suspect tooth. It might be fine, but it's not worth the risk of leaving it, in case it plays up in the next few months. I have to go back next Thursday to have the work done.

Next stop was my first visit to the oncology clinic. The reception area is lovely and made me feel very welcome. Andy came along with me to see my oncologist, who started by checking my wound, and he was happy that it was relatively clear of infection, enough so that my Portacath insertion can go ahead.

We then discussed all my treatment and what would happen. Each cycle starts a blood test two days before to make sure the blood count indicates I'm well enough for chemotherapy. Then chemotherapy follows, and the following day, I will have an injection to boost my immune system and help prevent infection.

I had a few basic questions I wanted answered.

"Should I have the flu jab?"

He said it's probably a good idea.

"Are probiotics safe during chemotherapy?"

Apparently there is no concrete evidence either way, so it's probably best to avoid them to make sure.

"What foods should I avoid during chemotherapy?"

Just be sensible with use by dates. I can have things like Blue cheese, which are at higher risk of causing problems, but in moderation.

"How do I avoid catching bugs?"

Keep a hand sanitiser near the front door and get people to use it. There is no need to be a hermit, and again, be sensible. Avoid people who are ill or have colds.

"Can I take multivitamins and use something like First Defence to help prevent colds?"

Yes, no problem at all.

"What painkillers can I take?"

Paracetamol, ibuprofen, and any of the usual ones.

This probably includes people dying of other causes. Without treatment, the survival rate is considerably less, and the effect of Herceptin is probably underestimated. The aim of treatment is to get cancer-free.

"Will I need a wig?"

Not everybody likes to wear one, but you will lose your hair, so you may want to be prepared.

"Can I travel abroad during treatment?"

Insurance costs make this prohibitive during treatment, and also, the risk of infection is very high.

After seeing the oncologist, we then met with one of the chemotherapy nurses who showed us around the chemotherapy suite and pointed out the complementary therapies area (each patient can have six complementary therapies and and usually book in on the day of blood tests).

Next week, I have a chemotherapy information appointment to find out more about my specific regime, and then will start chemotherapy soon after that.

My final appointment of the day was at a different hospital with the breast surgeon. He removed the dressings and agreed that I could proceed with the Portacath insertion tomorrow. I can also stop taking my antibiotics in 2 days, and the dressings can now stay off to let some air get to my wound so it can dry

16 FEBRUARY 2018

Andy has had to go to work, so his parents took me to the hospital for admittance for today's surgery. I had been on water only since 9:30 AM and I arrived at the ward for 1:30 PM. I was taken to bed 9, and I changed into a hospital gown. The doctor came to see me and explained the procedure: a small incision will be made near my collarbone for the port, which will be stitched in place just under the skin. The catheter will pass from the port into the jugular vein. There are some risks with it, and I was given the option of a PICC line instead, which is much simpler, but I would be left with the "tails" dangling down my arm, and it would be more susceptible to infection. I don't want something protruding from my skin, which will need changing from time to time, so I stuck with the plan of the Portacath, which can stay in place indefinitely.

A short while later, a nurse walked me down to the theatre. It was quite cold in the room, and there was a huge x-ray machine, which will be used to see my veins. Everyone was wearing protective clothing to shield them from the x-rays. I had a small step to stand on and climb onto the bed, which is much narrower than a standard hospital bed. Arm supports were inserted to keep my arms in place next to my sides, and the bed was raised slightly higher on the foot end. I needed a pillow under my knees as it pulled under my arm where I had the infection when fully extended with straight legs.

The doctor tried to insert a cannula so my sedative could be administered. He struggled to see any veins and then tried the back of my hand and inserted the cannula, but the vein collapsed, and it didn't work. A second cannula was then inserted in the crease of my elbow, and the first cannula was removed. There was a brief moment of excitement as blood sprayed from the successful cannula! As they plugged it and mopped up the mess, the doctor said, "Well, that one is working then!" Sheets were stuck to my chest and made into a shield over my face. I was given an oxygen mask, and I could now feel the warming pad underneath me, which kept me warm in the cold theatre. The sedative was admitted through an IV, and I was told I would start to feel a bit giddy and although I might be awake during surgery, with sedation, I wouldn't care what was done to me. Local anaesthetic was also injected, and wasn't long before I was oblivious to everything.

I woke up briefly as I heard metal tools clanking near my ear and then drifted off again for a while. When I woke up again, I could feel some tugging. "Just doing the last few stitches," said the doctor. I was now fairly awake, and I got very restless legs. Once all stitched internally, superglue was used instead of external stitches to seal the cut. Finally, they injected the port to flush it and check that it was working. The sheets were removed from my chest, and my oxygen mask was also removed. My bed from the ward was brought right up to the theatre bed, and I was asked to manoeuvre myself across so I could be taken back to the ward on my own bed. Once I was back in my cubicle and a bit more awake, I was brought a baguette, which I ordered from the sandwich list, along with my old favourite of fruit salad, which I find very satisfying when I'm in the hospital. Once I had eaten and been to the toilet, I was allowed to get dressed. The doctor popped in to see me briefly.

The Portacath felt very weird, like a muscle just before it cramps. The doctor explained that he had to put the catheter through the muscle, so that could be why. The port wasn't exactly where they planned, and it is a bit closer to my shoulder under my collarbone. Apparently, it is a bit trickier to place a Portacath on the left as you have to take a different path with the catheter. He has managed to leave a bit of length to stop the catheter wandering or moving. I was told I would probably feel a little bit stiff-necked for a couple of days, but I should get used to the strange sensation of the catheter in about a week.

I can shower tomorrow as the glue will have set enough to be waterproof by then, although I mustn't rub the area or try to clean it. I must just let the water run over it, although a bit of soap running over it won't do any harm. It was also suggested that I be careful when washing and don't go near the fresh wounds after cleaning where the infection was under my arm as we want to try and minimise the risk of cross-contamination. A little while later, I was discharged.

When I went to bed, my head was full of thoughts of my catheter coming loose and travelling into my heart. The thought of something going into my jugular vein was quite disturbing, and I imagined the vein ripping or bursting open if I moved too quickly. I also wondered what stops the bleeding as the catheter goes into the vein, and how big is the vain for the catheter to fit. The thoughts made me feel squeamish and were far worse than the actual discomfort from the procedure. I wasn't very comfortable in bed, and I felt a bit helpless being sore from surgery, as well the infection.

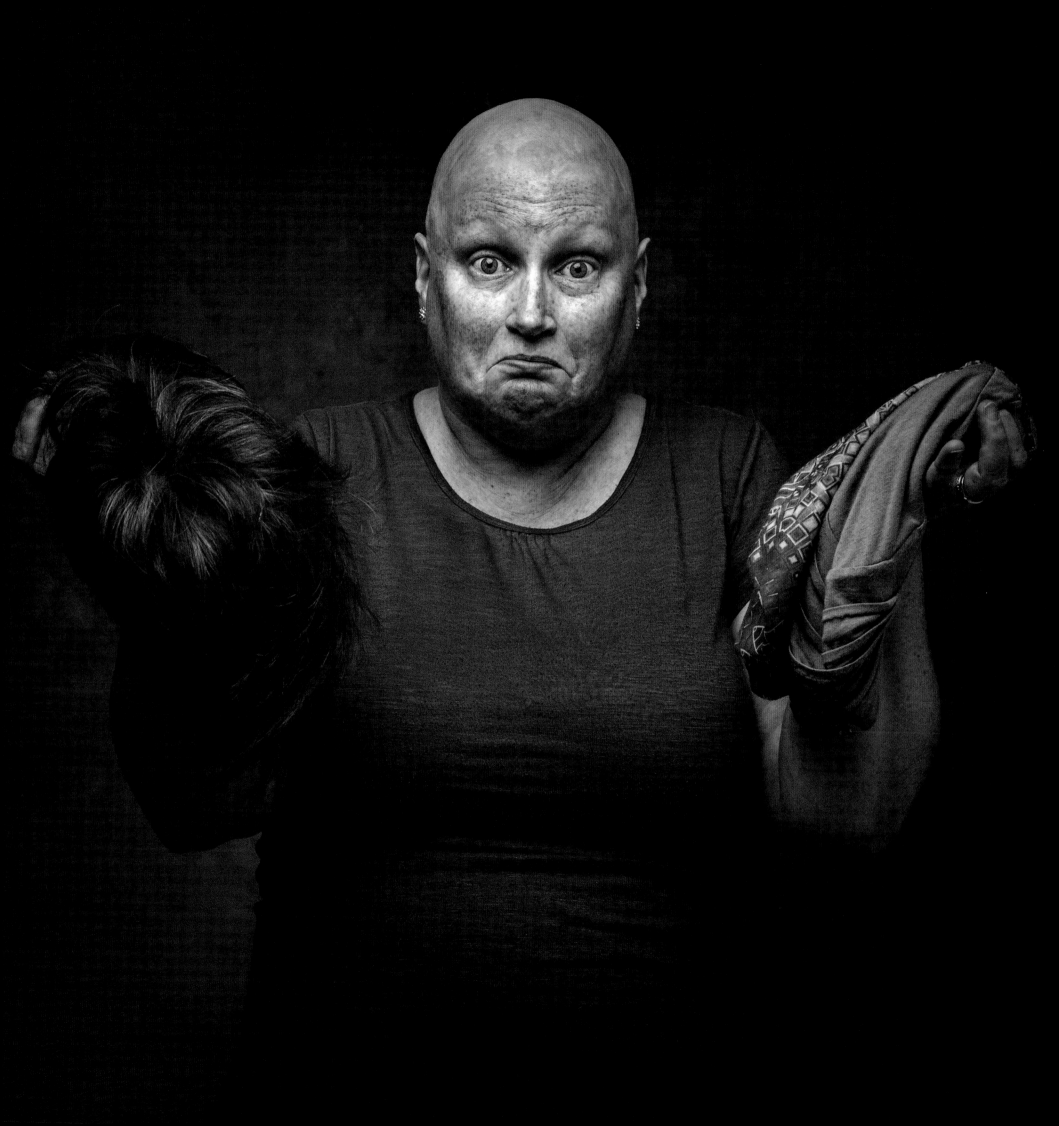

23 FEBRUARY 2018

The area where my Portacath was inserted is healing nicely. It was very itchy for a few days, and I resorted to taking an antihistamine. I think I might have had a reaction to the Dermabond glue, as it came up in a rash. Thankfully, it has settled down now, and is just a bit tender and bruised.

I have had a few appointments this week.

First was with the cardiologist — good news, I have a heart!

I had to have an echocardiogram, as Herceptin can damage the heart, so they need a baseline before any drugs are started. My heart was thoroughly scanned, and the images were fascinating. It was amazing to see and hear the blood pumping through the valves and chambers of your heart. You can actually see the valves opening and closing and the amplified sound, especially of the blood leaving the heart, sounds like rushing water. The clicks and pops from the various valves opening and closing reminded me of beatbox music. I wondered if anyone had created music from recorded heart sounds. I imagine it could be quite effective!

Thankfully, my heart is good and healthy and I will continue to have checks throughout my treatment to make sure it stays that way. Although Herceptin can damage the heart, if it is caught early, the Herceptin can be temporarily stopped to allow the heart to heal. If it is left, the damage can then become irreversible.

Yesterday, I went back to the dentist to have anything that could potentially cause problems checked and repaired. I had a filling replaced completely, one which was slightly under-filled, topped up, and a tooth in which I had root canal treatment over 30 years ago was reinforced. Using a special x-ray machine, I had a complete x-ray of my jaw and sinuses. I had to bite on a plate and was left alone in the room, and the machine started up and announced to me in an American accent, "your procedure will now begin…" As the plates revolved around my head, it played relaxing music, which for some reason made me want to laugh. The music stopped, and the computerised lady's voice told me, "your procedure is complete." She might actually have said, your operation is complete, as I remember thinking it was a slightly strange term for having an x-ray.

Today, I had my chemo information appointment. I was taken up to the chemotherapy suite and into one of the rooms where I had to sit in a very comfortable chair. I felt like I was on the throne, Queen of chemo! First, I had blood taken from my port. This is done by inserting a special needle with a gripper, through the skin, with a line attached like you have done to cannula, and they put a plaster over it to hold it in place. It was much easier than having to have a cannula inserted, and I'm so glad I opted to have a portacath. After my blood was taken, we went through my chemotherapy schedule from now until September, and radiotherapy will be added to that at a later date.

We then went over the different drugs and the common side-effects of them all.

Epirubicin will make my urine pink for about 48 hours. It will cause nausea, tiredness, mouth ulcers and hair loss.

Cyclophosphamide has the same side-effects, apart from the pink pee!

I will be given various anti-sickness drugs and steroids to counteract the worst side-effects. This is known as EC, and I will have four cycles every 21 days.

I was given details of complementary therapies, which are available to patients alongside chemo. The clinic also has well-being meetings once a month, so I will be well looked after.

26 FEBRUARY 2018

Today, I had a consultation for a wig. My friend Stefanie was coming along to offer her opinion on what suited me, but she then called to tell me she had a sore throat, so it wasn't worth the risk of passing an infection to me. She then suggested maybe we facetime so she could see the choices.

There was a wig selection for me to try. I decided to keep it short as it is short now, and many people think it suits me. Also, once I don't need to cover my bald head, I will have short hair as it grows, so I don't see the point of going back to long hair in the form of a wig.

We tried on a selection and narrowed it down to three. I FaceTimed Stephanie so she could see them on me. She didn't choose the one I fancied, but in the end, I actually liked the one she preferred best too.

To make the final decision, I kept all three for now, so I could show Andy and the girls. Andy was not bothered and doesn't mind which one I choose, but Caitlin hated them all. Hannah was on a skiing trip, so wasn't around to offer an opinion. I took some selfies to show some friends, and almost everybody picked the one that Stephanie chose, so I went with that.

27 FEBRUARY 2018

The worst snow for years in the UK known as the "Beast from the East" hit us and we woke up to 8 to 10 inches of snow. Thankfully, it was forecasted, and we thought to move the car onto the road just in case we couldn't get it off the drive. It was just a pity that someone, a.k.a., Andy, forgot to get fuel last night!

The appointment was at 10:30 A.M., and we gave ourselves plenty of time, leaving at 7:30 AM. We tried to head down to the main road to the petrol station, but it was down a steep hill with the sharp rise at the other end. It was a very slow and slippery journey, and we passed a few people walking. A man stopped us and said he got stuck and abandoned his car, and so had a lot of other people.

We decided to turn around and made it back up the hill. With the fuel gauge showing just 4 miles of fuel left, we crawled along, hoping to make it to the next petrol station. We merged into a stream of very slow-moving traffic (actually, mostly non-moving).

With 0 miles on the fuel gauge, we spotted the petrol station. I felt relieved as we crawled towards it, only to find it shut. The next petrol station was a few more miles away, and Andy now turned the car off every time we stopped to try and conserve fuel. Someone going in the opposite direction opened his window and told us the chaos was caused by a woman abandoning her car and creating contraflow. It took us an hour and a half to get the next mile or so down the road. It was very stressful worrying about the traffic, the lack of fuel, and the impending chemotherapy.

Finally, we made it to the petrol station. It was such a relief, at least we now knew we would make it. We continued to crawl into town and had a giggle as a man passed us on skis. I guess that is the best way to get around in this weather. Once we got into town, the roads were clearer, and we started to move. We made it to the coffee shop near the clinic in time for a quick drink before my appointment.

I was nervous about starting chemo, but also excited to start kicking cancer's butt!

The first drug was the "red devil," Epirubicin. I had a saline drip, and the red fluid was pushed into the line to my port from a large syringe. It was quite mesmerising to watch and reminded me of a lava lamp! I had two syringes of this and then two syringes of Cyclophosphamide. I also had anti-sickness medication and steroids. The steroids being injected caused the weirdest sensation in the most unexpected place! The nurse said to me, "you may get a little itch in your bottom". Next thing I knew, my eyes went wide and she laughed as I yelped and said, "I'll turn around if you want to scratch!" I suddenly felt like I was sitting on a sea urchin (having grown up in Cape Town, that was the first thing that came to mind) on reflection, it felt like someone had put stinging nettles in my knickers. It was the most peculiar, stinging, itching sensation right where I didn't want it!

I have further tablets to take at home for the next few days, as well as an injection in 24 hours, which will boost my immune system. With cycle 1 complete, we went out to lunch on the way home..

28 FEBRUARY 2018

So far, I 'm not feeling too bad, I am tired and feel a bit heady, but am okay. I was just a bit nervous about the injection I had to give myself, but I faced my fears and did it, and you know what? I hardly felt it! The fear was far worse than doing it. I set alarms for various times of the day to make sure I take all my medication at the right time.

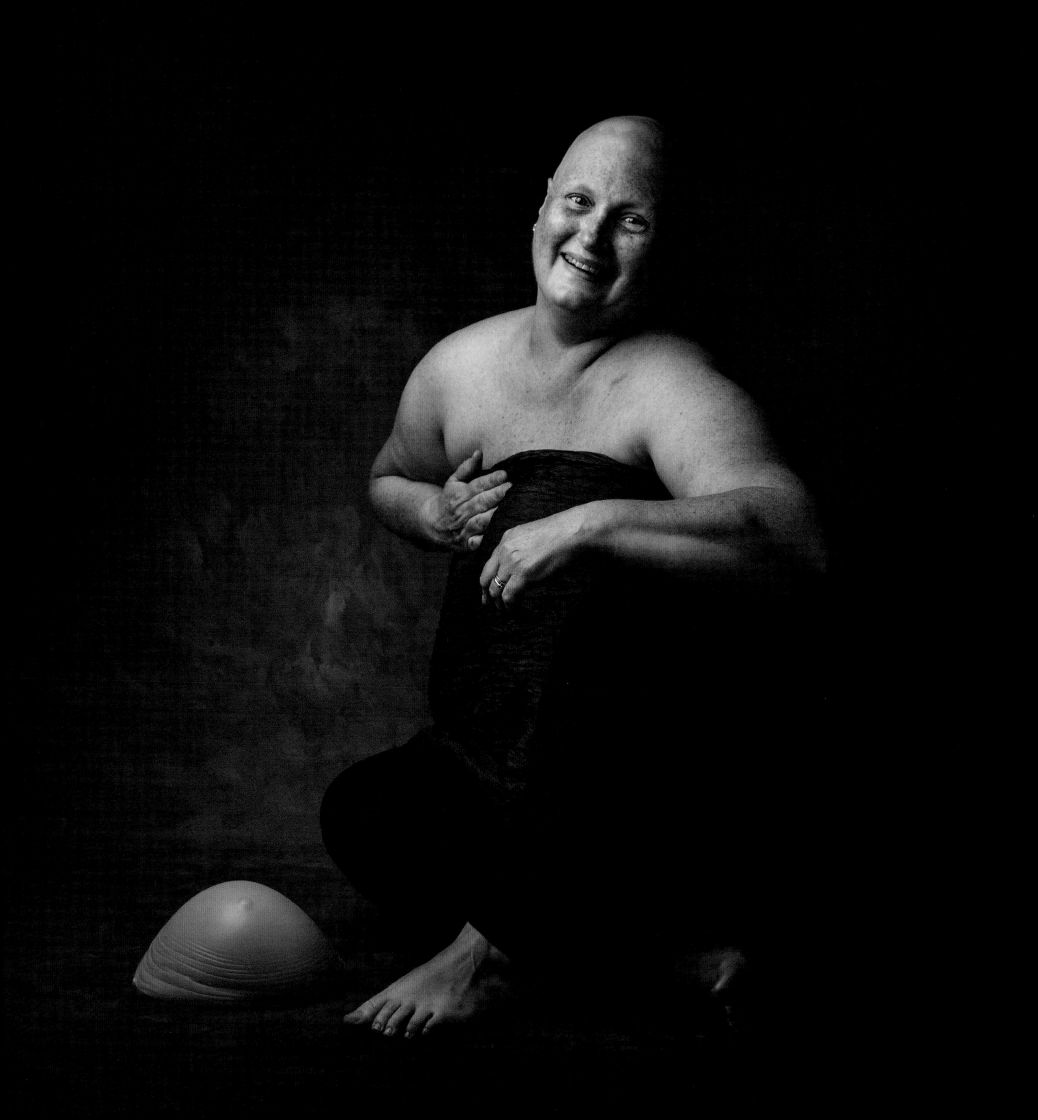

10 MARCH 2018

I haven't written anything for a while, but the chemo side-effects hit me like a ton of bricks. I have never felt so tired in my life – Real fatigue! I couldn't stay awake for more than 10 minutes at a time, and it was too much to even lift my mobile phone to check social media or play a game. I tried to watch TV in bed – I couldn't stay awake long enough – so I gave up. I felt a bit nauseous, but the anti-sickness drugs did the job for the most part. My taste buds have gone numb and I have a few ulcers in my mouth, but the mouthwash I was given tasted so bad that I would rather put up with the ulcers.

I started to feel better after the first week and managed to go out and do a few things.

We were out in the car this evening, and I ran my fingers on my hair, large chunks came out between fingers. I guess this was the start of my hair loss.

11 MARCH 2018

I've just found out that a fellow photographer and friend had been taken by this horrid disease! Alison had given me such strength since my diagnosis and been a great friend, offering me so much comfort in spite of her own suffering. We spoke about a day when we would both be well enough to meet up for a fun photo shoot together. Sleep sweetly, my beautiful friend.

13 MARCH 2018

My hair has been driving me insane; it was so sore and itchy. Andy did say he would shave it for me tonight when he gets in, but it was so uncomfortable that I had to get it done sooner. I couldn't wait any longer.

Crew cut is here! In desperation, I went to the hair salon where I had my hair cut short a couple of months ago. I went in wearing a hat to cover my hair loss. I told the hairdresser that I didn't want to watch it being cut, so she turned the chair away from the mirror, so I couldn't see what she was doing. I put my hat on again straight afterwards because I didn't want to look until I was at home on my own. I was rather surprised that she charged me to do it. You would think if you have been a paying customer before, then having to have your head shaved due to chemotherapy, they might do it free. Oh well, apparently not.

I am home now and built up the courage to look at myself in the mirror. It is very patchy where the hair was falling out in different amounts, and I look a bit like a dog with mange! I expected to look hideous, but it was not as bad as I thought, although it isn't exactly a pretty cut, and certainly not a look I would choose!

Andy knew today was a tough day for me, so he brought home a bottle of Prosecco for me. I was really touched by his thoughtfulness.

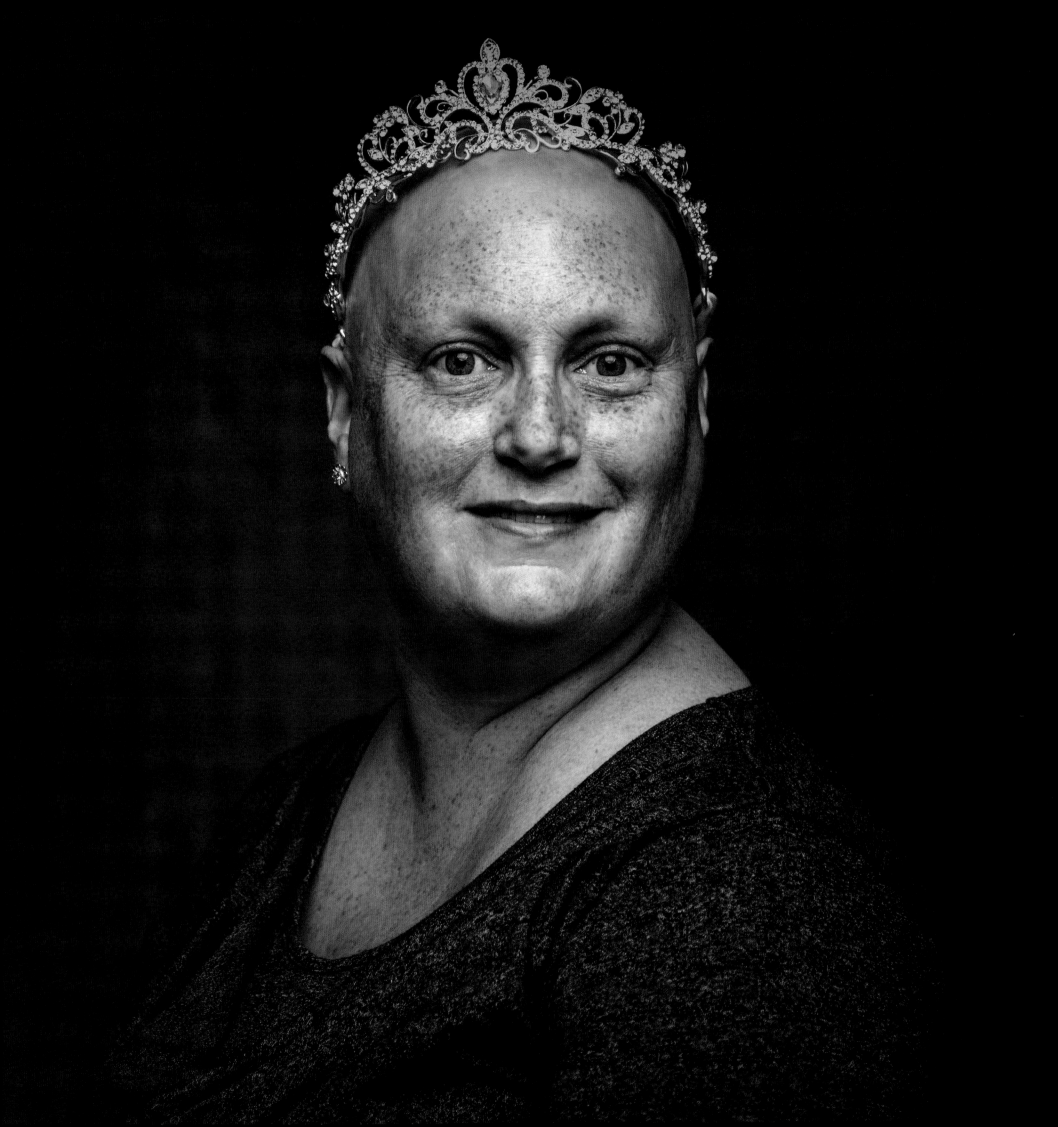

15 MARCH 2018

Even though I had a grade-one haircut, hair was still falling out everywhere. Tiny little hairs were getting on everything! It was quite annoying, but I'm so glad that I took control and cut, then shaved it. It would be so much more traumatic if I was losing my long hair. I am using Aloe Vera gel to sooth my scalp, as it is very sore and itchy.

Several people have asked me if I am trying a cold cap ("cold-capping" freezes the hair follicles and may slow down or limit the amount of hair which falls out), and I'm not. I decided that the fear and anticipation of losing my hair whilst trying to hold onto it by cold capping was worse than just facing the hair loss and getting on with it. I wanted to just take the plunge and get it over with, rather than living in the probably false hope of hanging on to it.

19 MARCH 2018

Tonight, there was a well-being evening at the clinic. I had my nails & eyelashes done, and a massage. I was also the model for the wigs. One thing I learnt is that I should never go blonde! It really doesn't suit me!

I have found the perfect solution to getting ready for a night out. You can save on washing your hair, drying your hair and even styling your hair. You can get ready in 2 seconds – you just need to go bald!

20 MARCH 2018

Gloves are off for round 2!

It was hard going back, knowing how bad the chemo made me feel the last time, and I was a bit depressed at the thought. I wanted to enjoy my weekend while I was feeling good, but I found it mentally difficult to cope, knowing I had to come back again! It was one thing going for it with complete ignorance; it was another having to do it knowing what was coming for the rest of the week!

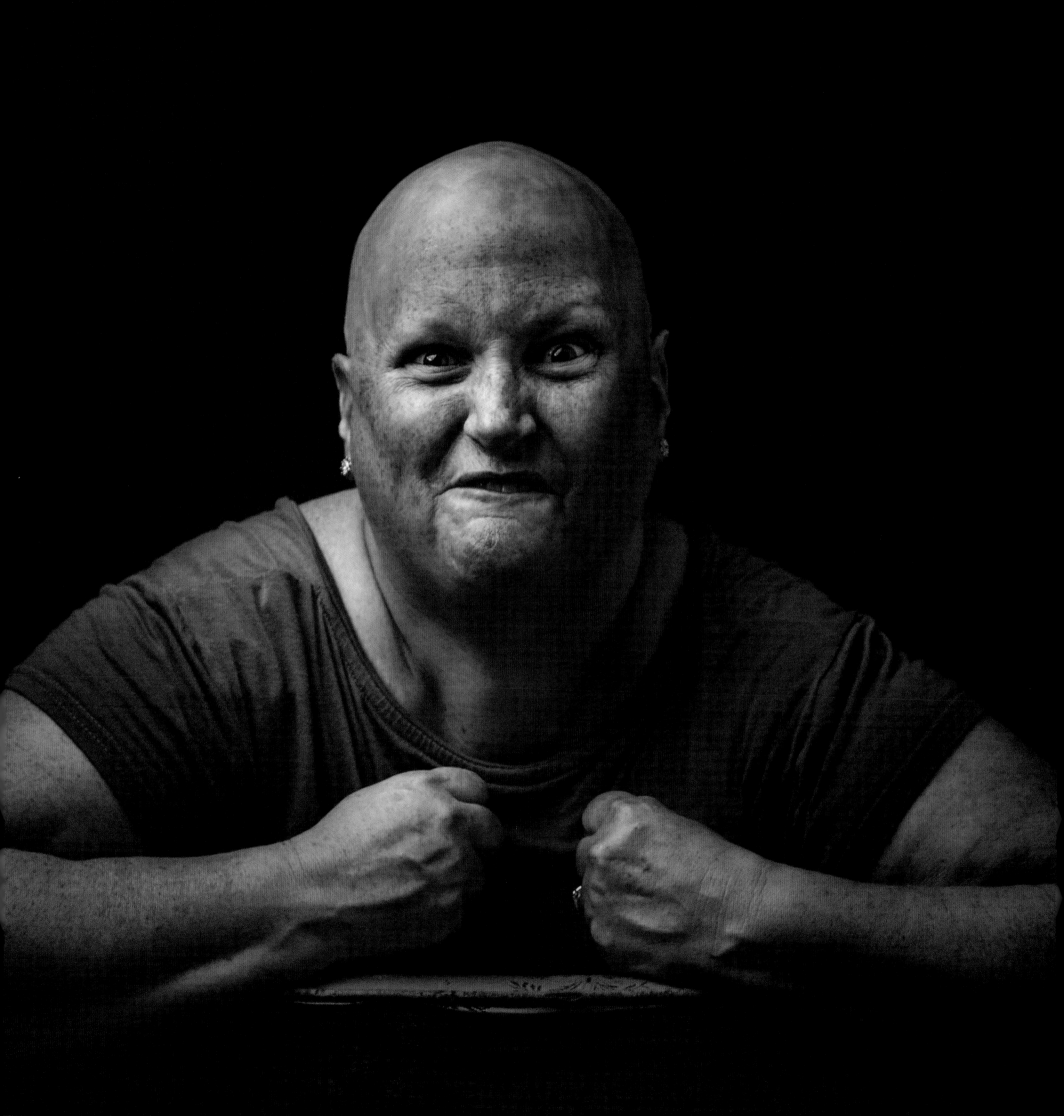

25 MARCH 2018

Everything has seemed very surreal, almost like I am outside my body and watching it happen to someone else. I've now lost most of the hair on my head, but being bald isn't as bad as I thought. It's certainly a lot quicker in the shower, and think of the savings on shampoo and conditioner! I'm well on my way to kicking cancer's butt, and I intend to do it with a smile on my face and positive thoughts in my head.

Yes, there are times that I feel awful, but I'm getting into a routine, and I'm trying to keep going with my photography. I've visited the rhinos that I love so much, and apart from a few days after chemo, I kept going. Some amazing people surround me, and I am fortunate enough to be part of the photographic community, which gives me tremendous strength. I have received so many beautiful cards and gifts from friends letting me know they are with me. I feel truly blessed to have such wonderful friends and family.

29 MARCH 2018

On the up from the chemo haze, it was pretty much the same as last time, but it is now 2 down and 2 to go of EC.

Andy now has more hair than I do for once in our lives. At least mine will grow back, though!

Most ladies can only imagine what they might look like bald. At least, that is one thing that's no longer a mystery to me! Looking for a positive here!

6 APRIL 2018

This morning, I went along to a MacMillan support group meeting where I met some lovely ladies at various stages of treatment. It was really good to meet up with other people going through something similar, and I think I will go every month, as long as treatment doesn't get in the way.

9 APRIL 2018

I went to the "Look Good, Feel Better" workshop today. It felt good to be in a room with so many other bald women! It was fun, and we got lots of makeup tips and a goody bag of lovely makeup to bring home.

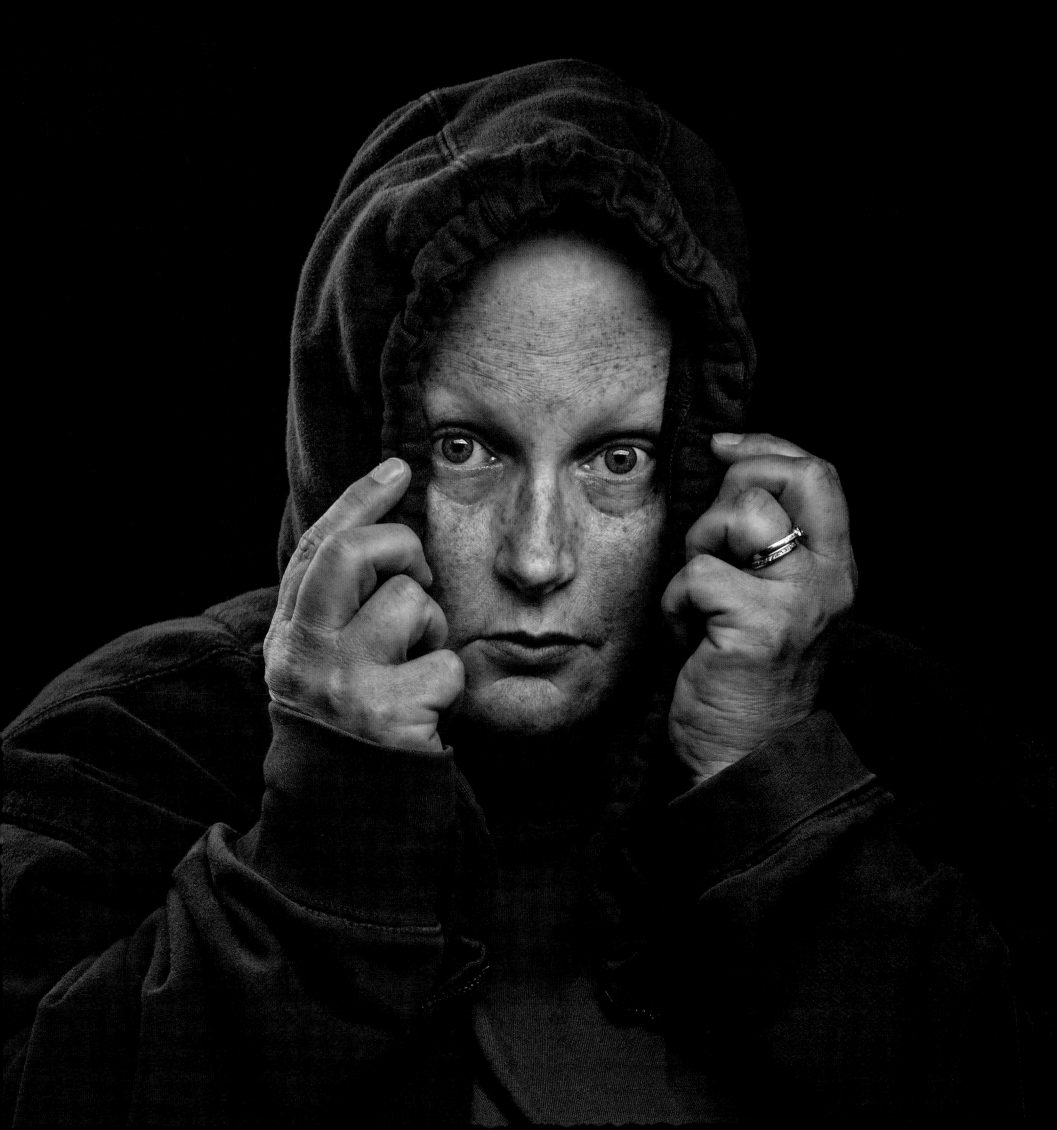

18 APRIL 2018

I think I can finally hold my camera again, so I have been in my studio taking self-portraits. I thought I should document my journey and take photos of myself at various stages of treatment.

19 APRIL 2018

I needed to get out of the house today in spite of feeling rough, so I went into the woods with Hannah this evening to take some photos of her. It was fun, but it really took it out of me. The walk back home was tough, and by the time we got in, I could hardly stand. Still, I got some lovely photos of her.

24 APRIL 2018

I went back into my studio today and took some more self-portraits. I wanted to get one of me crying, so I made myself think of something very sad, and it worked. I remembered a song that makes me think of my brother who died when he was 19 and I ended up sobbing and pushing the remote trigger on my camera. I got some seriously ugly photos of myself, and it was emotionally draining. Hope I sleep well tonight after that!

4 MAY 2018

The latest Cameracraft (an international photography magazine) came out today, and I was featured in it as one of 3 award-winning female photographers. Not only that, my image was on the cover! I was beyond delighted. I think I did a little dance when the postman arrived with it.

5 MAY 2018

The best way I can think of how to describe the way I feel today would be understood by any Harry Potter fan! I think the dementors are attacking me and have sucked the life out of me. I can't wait for chemo to be over!

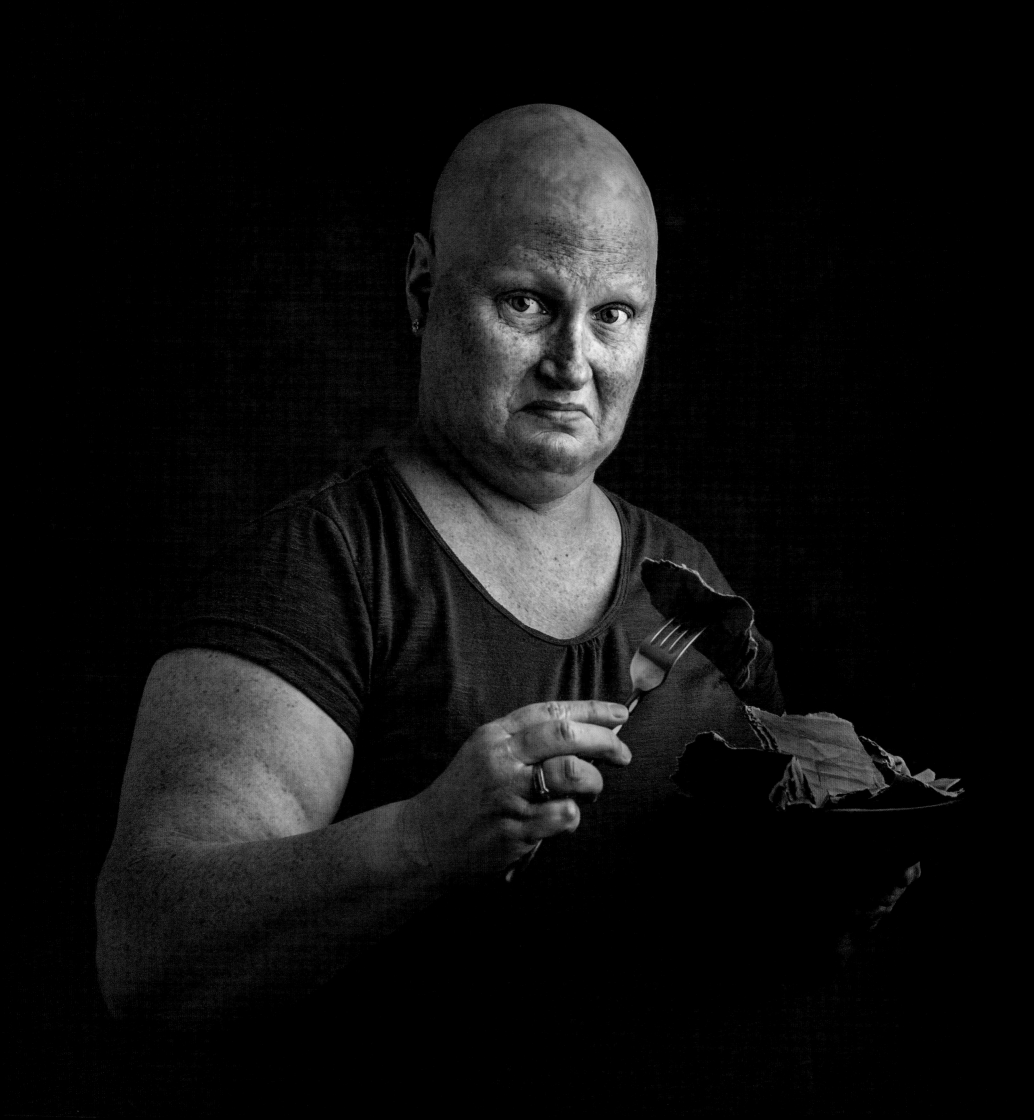

7 MAY 2018

Each cycle of EC has been pretty much the same. I've been sick a couple of times with each cycle, but I coped. Having no taste has been pretty depressing. I would feel hungry, then wouldn't know what I fancy or what will make me feel better, and I've got down about that a few times. I am completely off cheese — it tastes revolting! I don't want alcohol or chocolate either, and I have a typical "moon face" from the steroids. It was a beautiful bank holiday weekend and I was feeling weak, but well enough to sit in the garden on the swing seat and enjoy the weather.

8 MAY 2018

It was so hard to sleep. I felt so miserable, and my mouth was sore, like it was full of cotton wool. I got up at 3 a.m. and got an ice-lolly from the freezer (they are about the only thing I can stand to eat) and went into the lounge. I did laugh at myself in spite of feeling so rough. The new garden egg chair was in the lounge (until it is warm enough to go outside), and it is quite comforting to swing in it. There I was, completely naked, swinging in a garden egg chair in the living room while eating an ice-lolly at 3 a.m.! Only a cancer patient would get away with that!

12 MAY 2018

My beautiful friend, Amanda, is walking tonight, in her bra, for cancer in the London Moonwalk. I wish her all the luck in the world. She has got my name on her sweatshirt with some other people she knows who are either fighting or have had cancer. She has kept me going with her posts and support and has been such an inspiration. You go, girl!

14 MAY 2018

I made it to the Newborn Photography Show. Yay! I was going to wear my wig to the awards evening, but I left it at home. People have been encouraging and said to embrace the bald and just wear something on my head. I walked around with a large flower crown over my hat today for a laugh. I would have been way too embarrassed to do that before cancer, funny how it changes you.

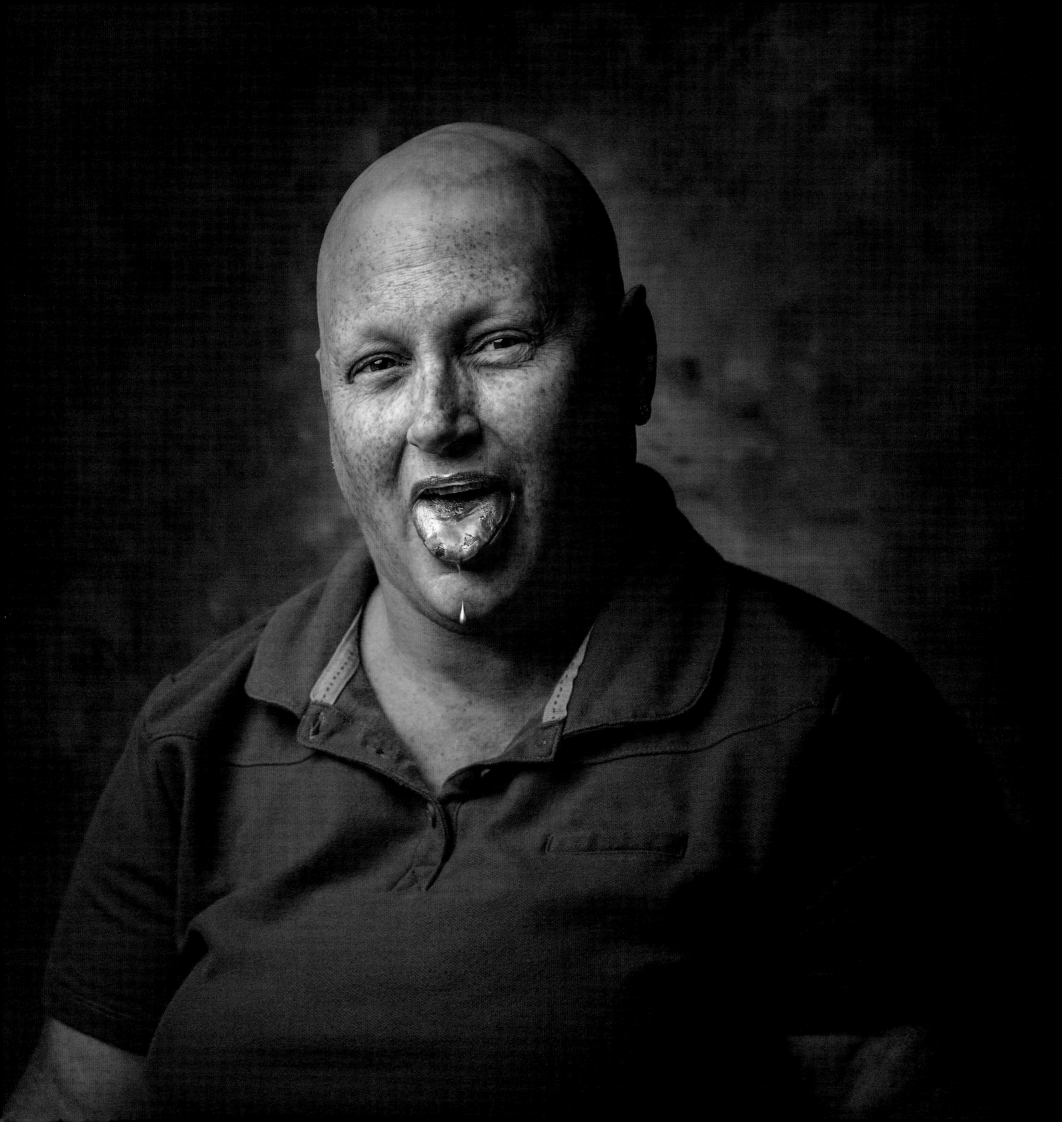

16 MAY 2018

I went to put on makeup for the evening. Thing is, when you are bald and have no hairline, how do you know where to stop with your foundation? I could just keep going all the way round until I get to the back of my neck!

I had such fun with friends, and I did embrace my baldness! I bought a tiara from one of the traders and went to the dinner with a bald head on display and the tiara perched on my shiny scalp.

When we sat down for dinner, the music started, and the first song was "This is Me" from the Greatest Showman. It suddenly struck me, while I was sitting there with my bald head and tiara, listening to the words, "I am brave, I am bruised, this is who I'm meant to be..." how poignant the moment was, and the tears started flowing down my cheeks. They were happy and satisfied tears as I realised that this is my life and I need to make the most of it! Everybody made me feel so comfortable. I felt like a princess, and it was such fun to just let go and dance and forget about cancer for the night!

17 MAY 2018

I saw my oncologist today, and everything is going well. I chatted about my photographs, and he thinks they will make a wonderful set of images. He asked if I had photographed other people. I haven't yet, but I am going to try and get other people to photograph in my studio to show their emotions and side effects that go with cancer. He said it was ok for me to put up a poster in the clinic asking people if they wanted to participate in the project, which I ghave called "Faces of Cancer."

22 MAY 2018

First, Herceptin! It's a subcutaneous injection, which takes about 5 minutes, but it stings like hell! It feels like a wasp sting. I've got to stay for 6 hours in case I have an allergic reaction. At least, they feed us. There is a lovely menu from which we can choose sandwiches freshly made to order.

It was a long day, but at least I didn't have any reaction to Herceptin. Next time, they need to monitor me for just 2 hours after the injection.

23 MAY 2018

New chemo regime - Paclitaxel.

It's quite scary changing drugs; I hope it isn't as bad as EC. This is a much longer infusion, which takes 3 hours. It is covered with a black bag, as it is sensitive to light. It is given with a high dose of antihistamine, and I was told that for the next 24 hours, I must not operate any wheeled equipment, not even the wheelie bin!

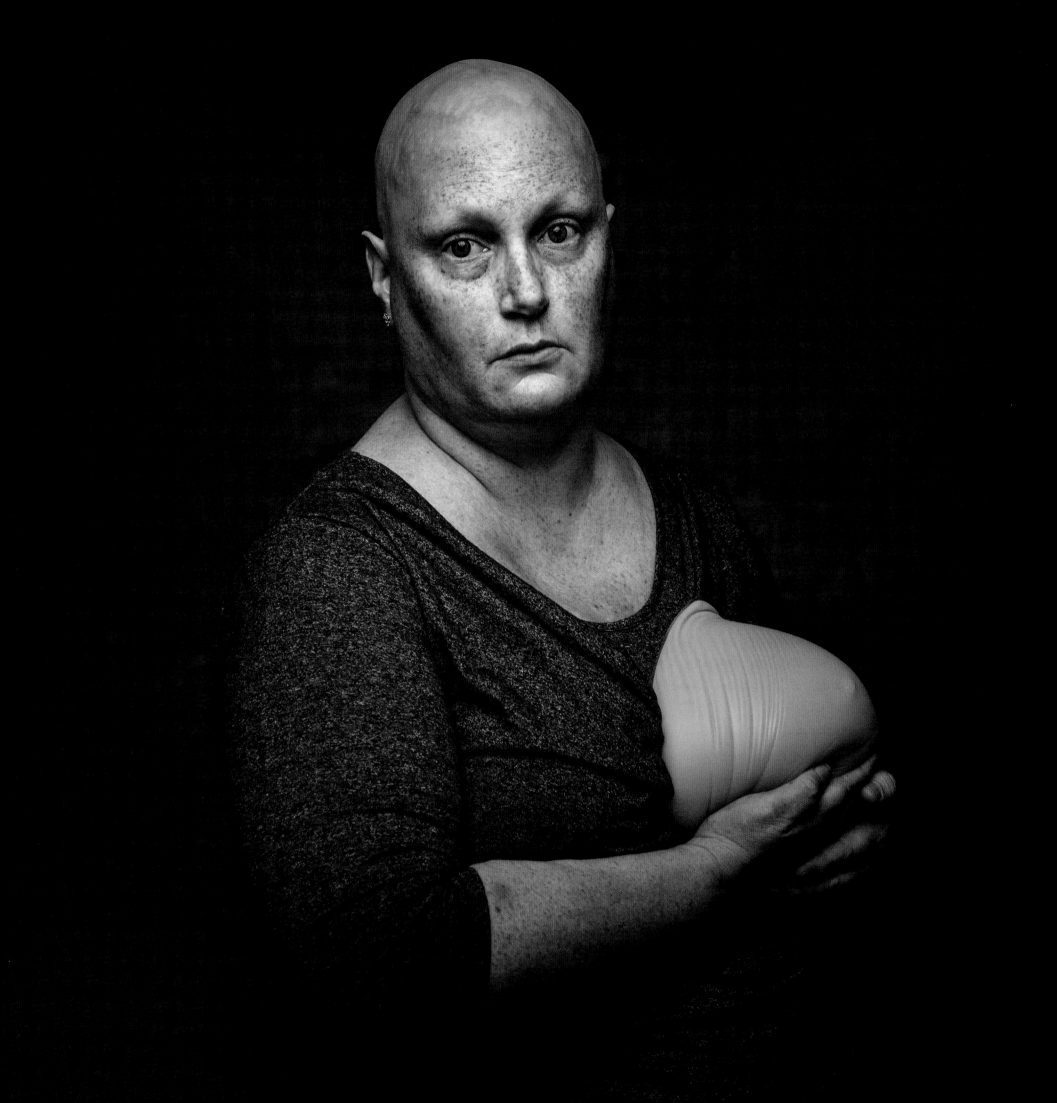

24 MAY 2018

So far, I feel okay, but the nurse did tell me not to be led into a false sense of security, as it could take a few days for the effects of the drugs to be felt, especially after the steroids leave my system.

27 MAY 2018

Paclitaxel is not nice! I am in so much pain. I can hardly walk. My head feels a lot clearer than it did with EC, but I am so uncomfortable. Just walking to the kitchen, I have to hang onto the walls, as it feels like my legs are going to buckle under me. I have got the worst restless legs, and I can't sleep!

I have neuropathy in my fingers and toes, so they feel numb and tingly, so my oncologist has decided to reduce the dose, to reduce the risk of the neuropathy lasting beyond treatment.

30 MAY 2018

Still struggling after my Paclitaxel, but I had my first person in today for a shoot for Faces of Cancer. I was nervous, but excited.

It went really well, he was amazing. It was a man called Stuart, who had breast cancer and has had a mastectomy. We spent so much time talking and then took photos. I was really pleased with the outcome and can't wait to do more for the project!

1 JUNE 2018

I am really aching, but it was the MacMillan support group this morning, and I felt that if I went and had a chat with everyone, it would cheer me up and take my mind off how I am feeling. I am really lucky and very grateful to have a support group, and the bonus is lovely cake and coffee.

5 JUNE 2018

After seeing my oncologist, my dose of Paclitaxel was reduced to 75%, due to the neuropathy. If it gets too bad, then it could last for up to 18 months, and I don't want numb fingers for that length of time! Today, I will have the lower dose, but it still takes 3 hours to infuse!

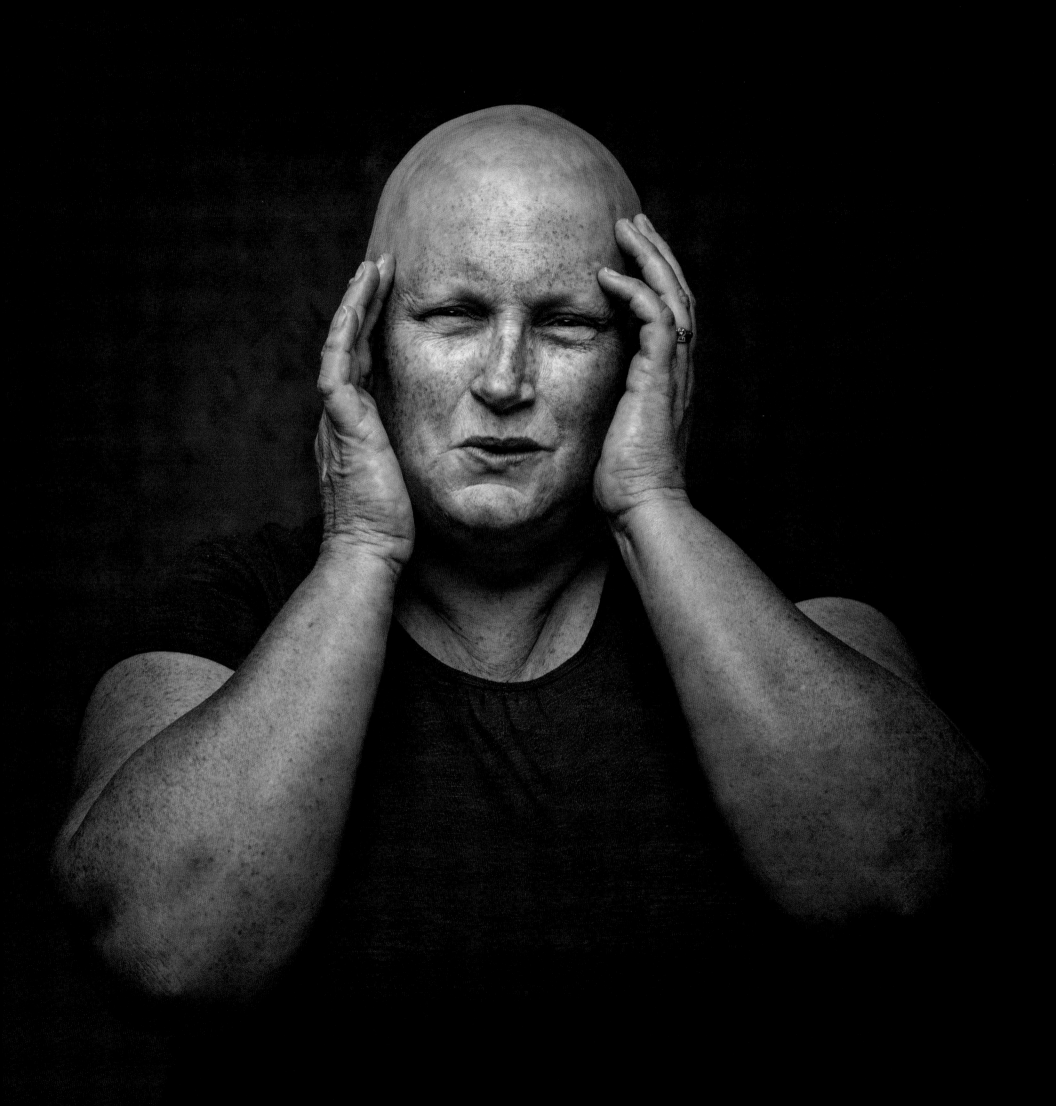

10 JUNE 2018

All through my chemotherapy, I have had a huge urge to have my feet in the sand with the waves washing over them. I did that today. I had a really bad night and couldn't sleep at all. I am still very uncomfortable on Paclitaxel, but with the reduced dose, the pain isn't nearly as bad! The sea felt so good on my feet; I didn't want to leave!

19 JUNE 2018

Second to last chemo.

I've been achy and uncomfortable, but I've still been doing things. I don't feel sick at all, and I no longer feel like my head is in a bubble.

Chemo ate my eyebrows! My eyebrows and eyelashes have finally fallen out, which makes me look really ill!

20 JUNE 2018

I took the plunge and entered self-portraits into the London & Essex region Master Photographers Association annual print competition. I was so nervous to show vulnerable pictures of myself!

It was a great evening though, and I not only won the portrait category and took 2nd place, I was also named overall Photographer of the Year for the region. I am so happy!

27 JUNE 2018

I can't believe that today is my dad's 95th birthday! Wow, how amazing to get to that age. I wonder how old I will be when I die. Cancer has a way of making your look at your life and mortality!

3 JULY 2018

Last chemo! Yay! I can't believe I have got here!

I spotted myself in the bathroom mirror this morning, and I couldn't decide if I looked more like Mr Blobby, Lord Voldemort, or the comedian, Harry Hill! None of them is a great look for a woman.

6 JULY 2018

Cake and coffee again today at the Macmillan support group at the hospital. I've made friends with people in the group now, so I looking forward to catching up.

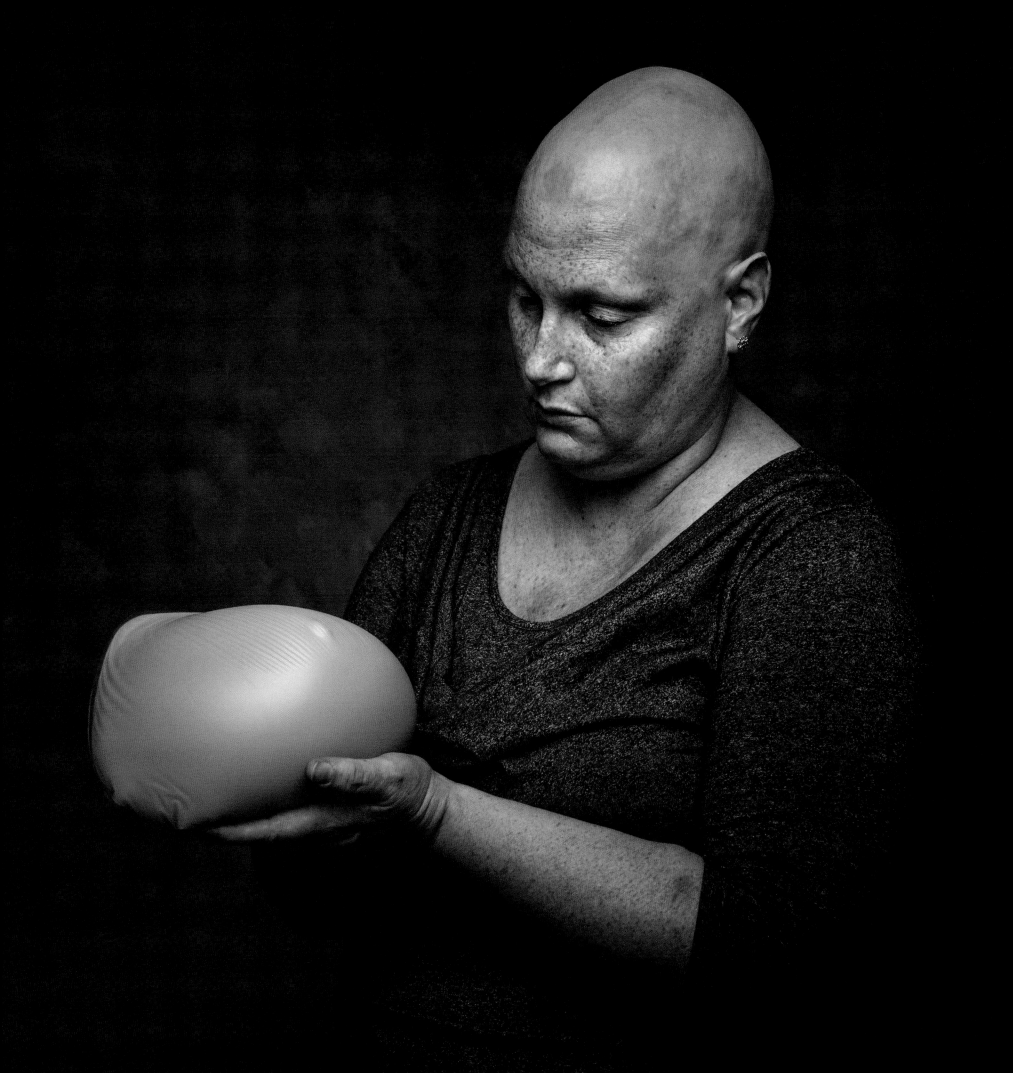

11 JULY 2018

My oncologist has been telling lots of people about my photos. I had an email today from a doctor at Guy's Hospital. She asked if she could use my images for teaching, "As they are striking and say so much about the experience of cancer, without needing any accompanying words." Of course, I said yes! I want them to help people.

16 JULY 2018

I was invited to exhibit some of my Faces of Cancer portraits at the Breast Cancer Kent's Awards this evening. It was a great night, and I received some wonderful feedback on my images!

24 JULY 2018

I just had my first tattoo!

Well, I had a CT scan in preparation for radiotherapy. I changed into a hospital gown on my top half. There was only one hanging up in the changing room, and it was a bit tight (well, more than a bit). I squeezed into it as best I could (Thank goodness I only have one boob, or I would never have got it on!).

Once I was in the room, I had to unbutton it anyway and have the scan. After the scan, they made 3 tiny pinpricks and gave me my radiotherapy tattoos. I have one in the middle of my chest and one on each side, so I can be lined up each time I have radiotherapy.

It was quite amusing posting on Facebook that I had my first tattoo and seeing the reactions from everyone.

26 JULY 2018

My friend's son had his head shaved today to raise money for Cancer Research. He said he wanted to do it not long after my diagnosis, but he had to wait until the school holidays. His school was not very supportive, and his mum was told that he will be excluded from school if his hair hasn't grown back to at least a grade 3 by the time he goes back in the Autumn. I can't believe that attitude. You would have thought they would support him as it's for a good cause.

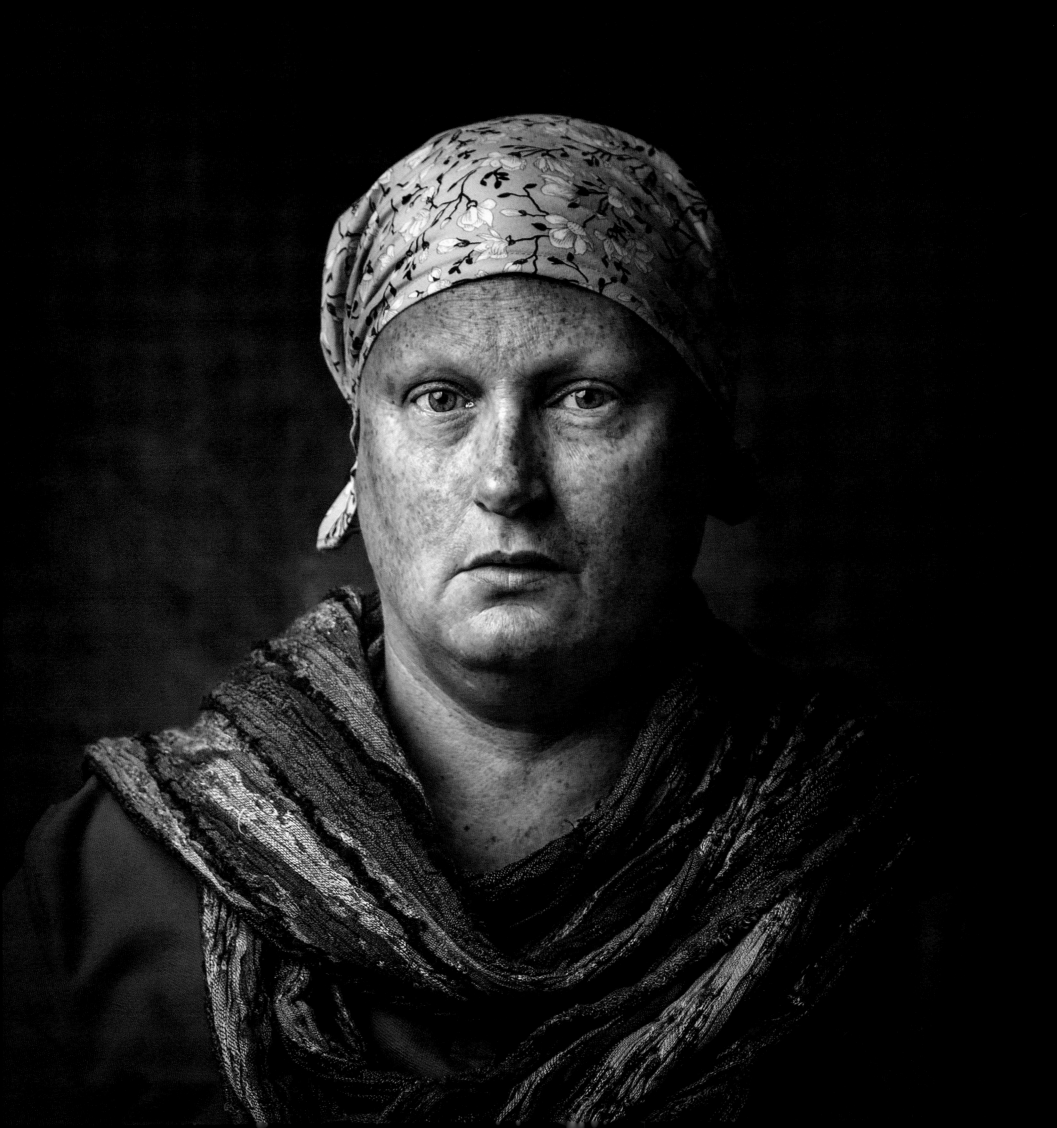

8 AUGUST 2018

I started radiotherapy today. I now have to go to the clinic every working day for 15 days in a row. Talk about tedious.

I changed my top half into a gown and had my palm scanned as identification, which will be done each time, and then had to lie down on the bed with my arms above my head. There were supports for my wrists, so I knew where to put them. The light was blue and black (almost like a huge QR code) and the radiographers lined me up precisely using my tattoos as markers to get me into the correct position. I had to keep completely still and they left the room. An alarm sounded to warn people of the radiation, and the machine started to move around me. I was not enclosed in any way and could clearly see the machine and the ceiling. As the machine moved, I could see the metal plates moving to create the shape of the area to be radiated. There was a green light, and then a noise as the radiation beam was fired at me. The machine then moved and the plates realigned for the next part of my body. This happened 3 times, and that's it. It's not scary and doesn't hurt.

14 AUGUST 2018

Herceptin 5 of 18 today, and radiotherapy 5 or 15.

All good with radiotherapy so far. My skin is just changing colour slightly, and you can see a line where the radiation has been.

21 AUGUST 2018

I had another request today to use my images, this time, by a breast cancer charity. They are starting to be noticed, and I have had a few people message or email to ask about using them.

26 AUGUST 2018

I have just noticed that my eyelashes and eyebrows are growing back. I have a tiny little line of short eyelashes. It looks funny, but they are on their way!

29 AUGUST 2018

Last session of radiotherapy!

It's actually gone quite quickly. I can't believe that all the worst treatments are over! I have blistered slightly and have a rash from the radiation, but it was relatively easy compared with what I have already been through.

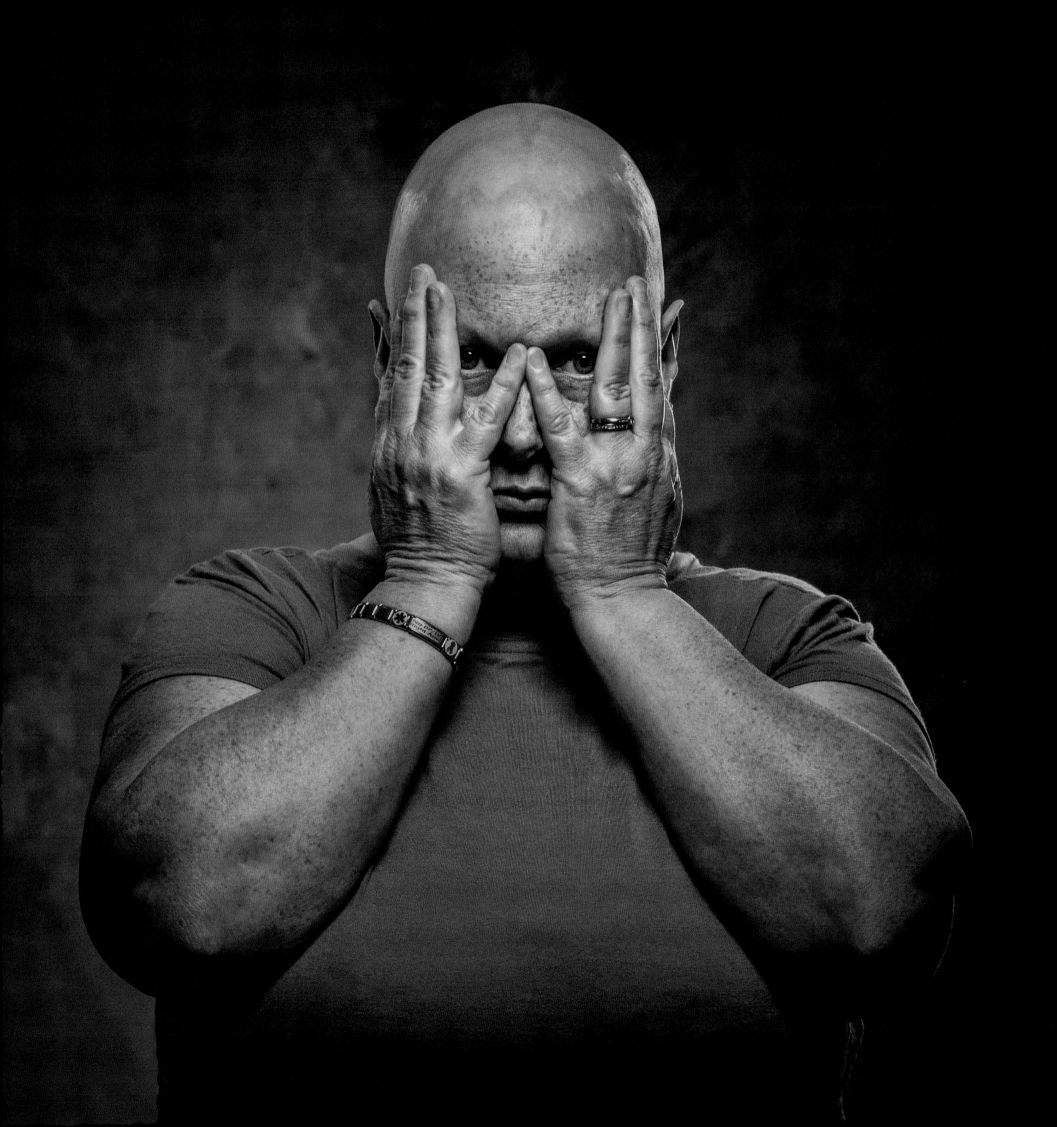

12 SEPTEMBER 2018

I have now photographed 22 other people and yesterday, I drove up to Darlington to the headquarters of the Master Photographers Association. This morning, a selection of 20 of the images was submitted to a panel of world-renowned judges to be considered for an associate qualification. I walked into the room once judging was complete to be told the outcome. The chairman of qualifications walked over and said to me, "I am afraid we have not been able to award you your associateship today…" It seemed like time slowed down as I wondered where I had gone so wrong, when he continued, "we have decided to award you with a fellowship instead."

There were tears all around, and I still can't believe it. I was stunned and delighted that the judges deemed it worthy of an upgrade and awarded me a Fellowship with the Master Photographers Association. Fellowship of the MPA is a very difficult qualification to achieve within the photographic profession, as this takes a great deal of time, work and dedication to your art to reach this level. Only 1% of photographers achieve this level.

I was amazed when one of the world's top photographers and international judge, Trevor Yerbury, posted the following on Facebook;

> "I have judged many A&F qualification panels over the years for several photographic bodies, but there are always a few, very few, that will forever remain in your mind.
>
> Today was one of those rare moments when a panel for an 'A' qualification was judged. After a couple of minutes viewing the images, I simply replaced my score pad and said to my fellow judges, 'I cannot even begin to take marks away from such a stunning and emotional body of work.' My fellow judges were in total agreement, and following a brief discussion, we all agreed that we should award the author a Fellowship of the Master Photographers Association – such was the impact her work had on us all.
>
> Thank you to my fellow judges and Chair of Qualifications for their support, and if you ever get to view this work, I implore you to take the opportunity. It was a very emotional moment, and a few tears were shed! Many, many congratulations to Imelda Bell. This is what real photography can do."

Trevor's equally renowned wife, Faye, who is also a world-class photographer and judge, shared the images, saying the following;

> "Sharing one of the most incredible panels of work I have ever been invited to judge for the assessment of Associateship. It was so well put together, thought out, and as creative as I have ever witnessed. The photography for close-up portraiture and the quality of the presentation meant that as we looked at one another on the team, we just had to resubmit it as a FELLOWSHIP, and that is exactly what Imelda was awarded with.
>
> Congratulations, Imelda, and I hope you give many photographers the inspiration to do what you have done. Simplistic and beautiful photography made a wonderful collection of images."

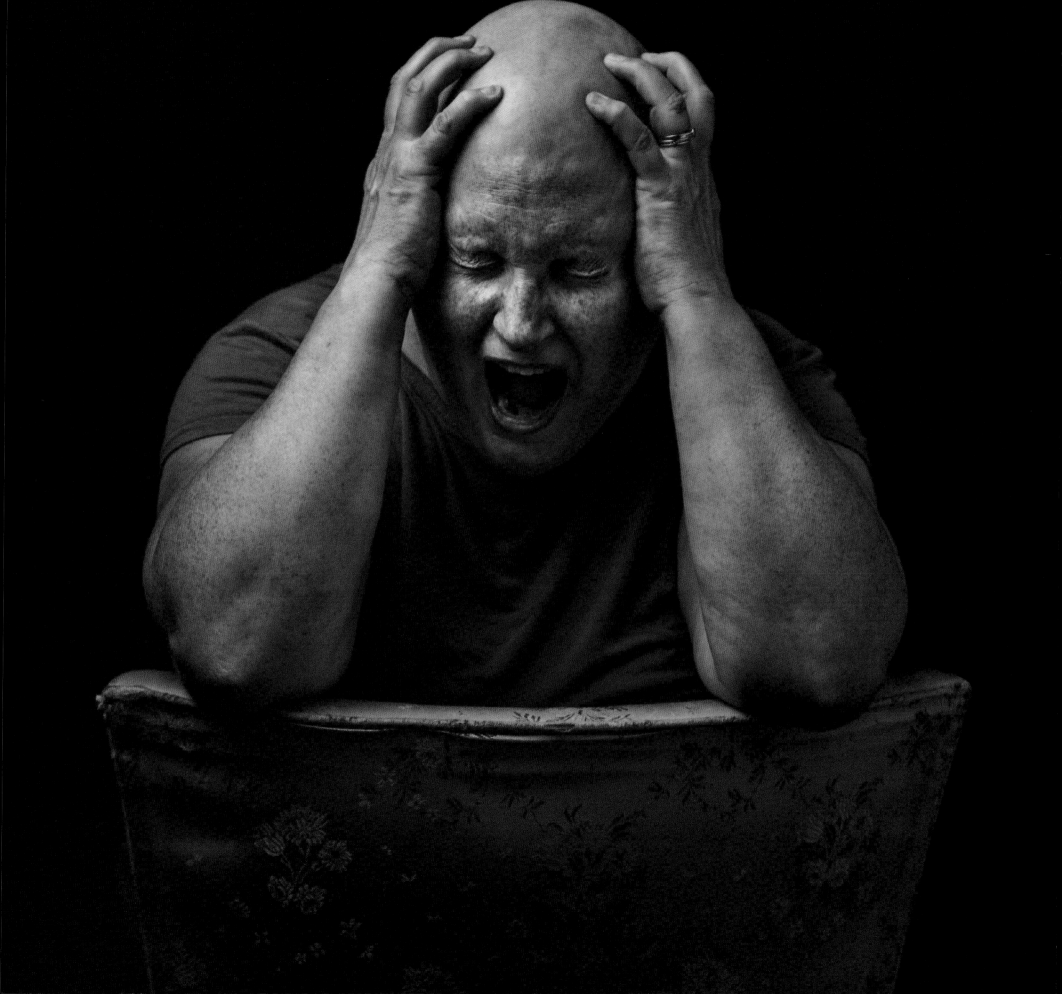

7 OCTOBER 2018

I've been at the MPA awards this weekend, and I won the best fellowship in 2018. I can't believe how this year has turned around for me.

The chairman of the MPA commented, "You have now achieved the greatest accolade possible to any photographer, the BEST Fellowship panel of the year, that stands head and shoulders above anything else you will ever do (except beating the big C). You are now standing at the very top; your future is to help to pull others up behind you, you cannot go higher with other little insignificant awards, you can only strive to improve and inspire others..."

That is what I want to do with "Faces of Cancer" – inspire not only other photographers, but to help people affected by Cancer, through my imagery, to see that we can continue to live and enjoy life, and although there are scary and dark times, there are also times of happiness, tremendous love, and laughter. The aim of my series of images (of which there are now over 60 including about 40 self-portraits) is to help people to see that there is still life with cancer, even if it is terminal.

8 OCTOBER 2018

I arrived home this evening and received a very sad message. Less than 24 hours since I was presented with the award, one of the people in my panel passed away. Scott was very proud to appear in this body of work, and I was honoured to have got to know him. I want to dedicate my win to Scott, and I hope that his portrait, along with the others I have created, will help people throughout the world to deal with cancer.

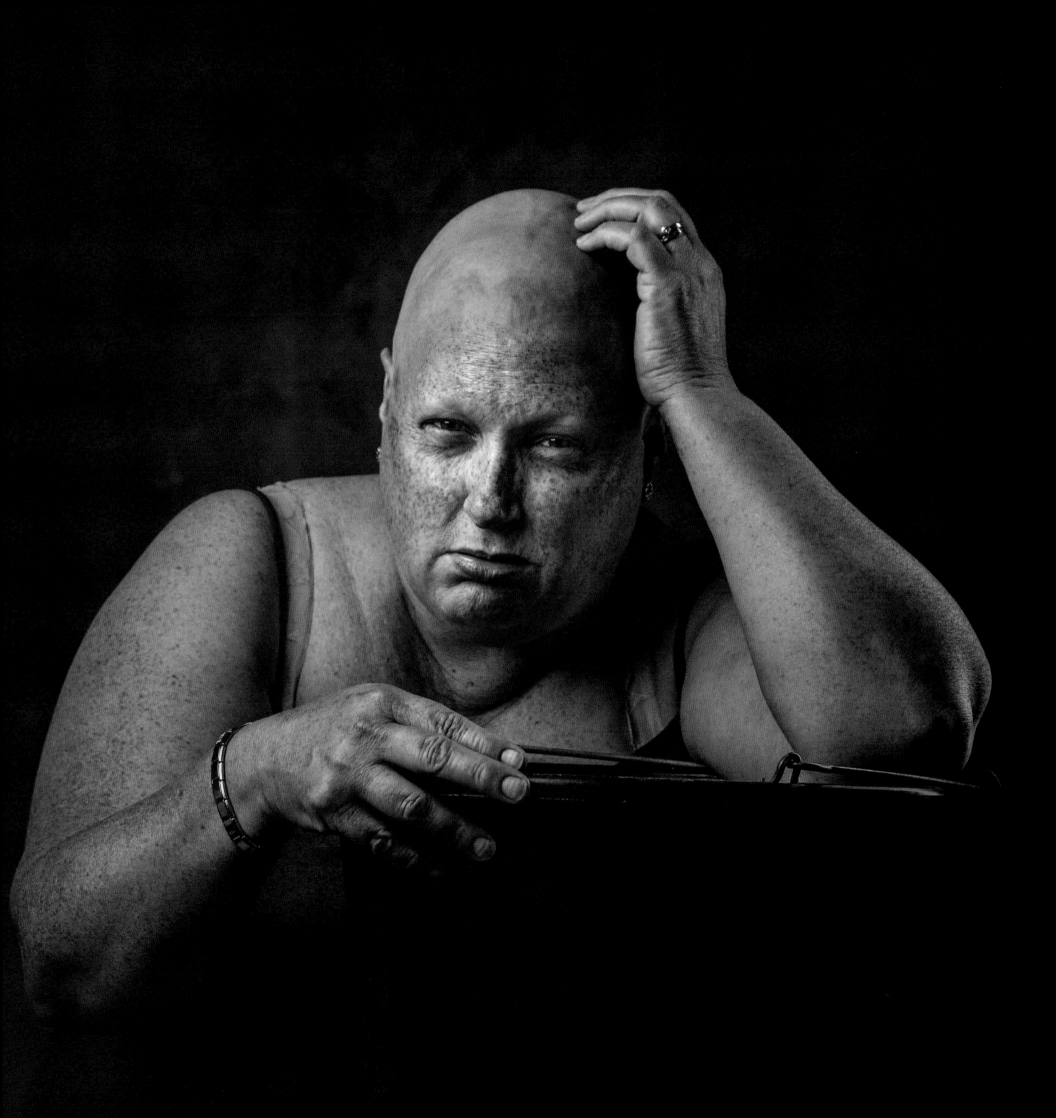

2 NOVEMBER 2018

At each of the support group meetings, we have a different speaker. We have had talks on relaxation, anxiety, exercise and lots of other things. Today's talk was really fascinating.

We had some ladies from the charity Medical Detection Dogs come to speak to us. It's amazing how man's best friend is helping so many people. Dogs are trained as medical alert assistants to support people with complex health conditions like diabetes, epilepsy and severe nut allergies. Using their sense of smell, the dogs detect tiny odour changes emitted prior to an emergency and lets the person take preventative action. This helps reduce paramedic callouts and hospital admissions; giving people and their families greater confidence and independence to lead full, happy lives.

Other dogs are trained as bio-detection dogs, and they detect the minute odours associated with many cancers in breath or urine samples, as well as other diseases like Parkinson's and malaria (which is detected in sweat in socks). It is pioneering work which could help scientists develop faster, cheaper, non-invasive methods of diagnosis.

Recently, one of the dogs, Freya, was flown out (business class, of course) to the Massachusetts Institute of Technology (MIT) to help with their development of the "e-nose". Research is still in its early stages, but it is a possibility in the future. Current e-noses are about as good as ours, but "they're not as good as a dog's nose, which is anywhere from 10,000 to 100,000 times as acute as our own."

I found the whole morning really interesting. As an animal lover, I love it when animals and humans work together in a loving and healthy way.

I have found the support group so helpful, and I intend to keep going through the remainder of my treatment and beyond.

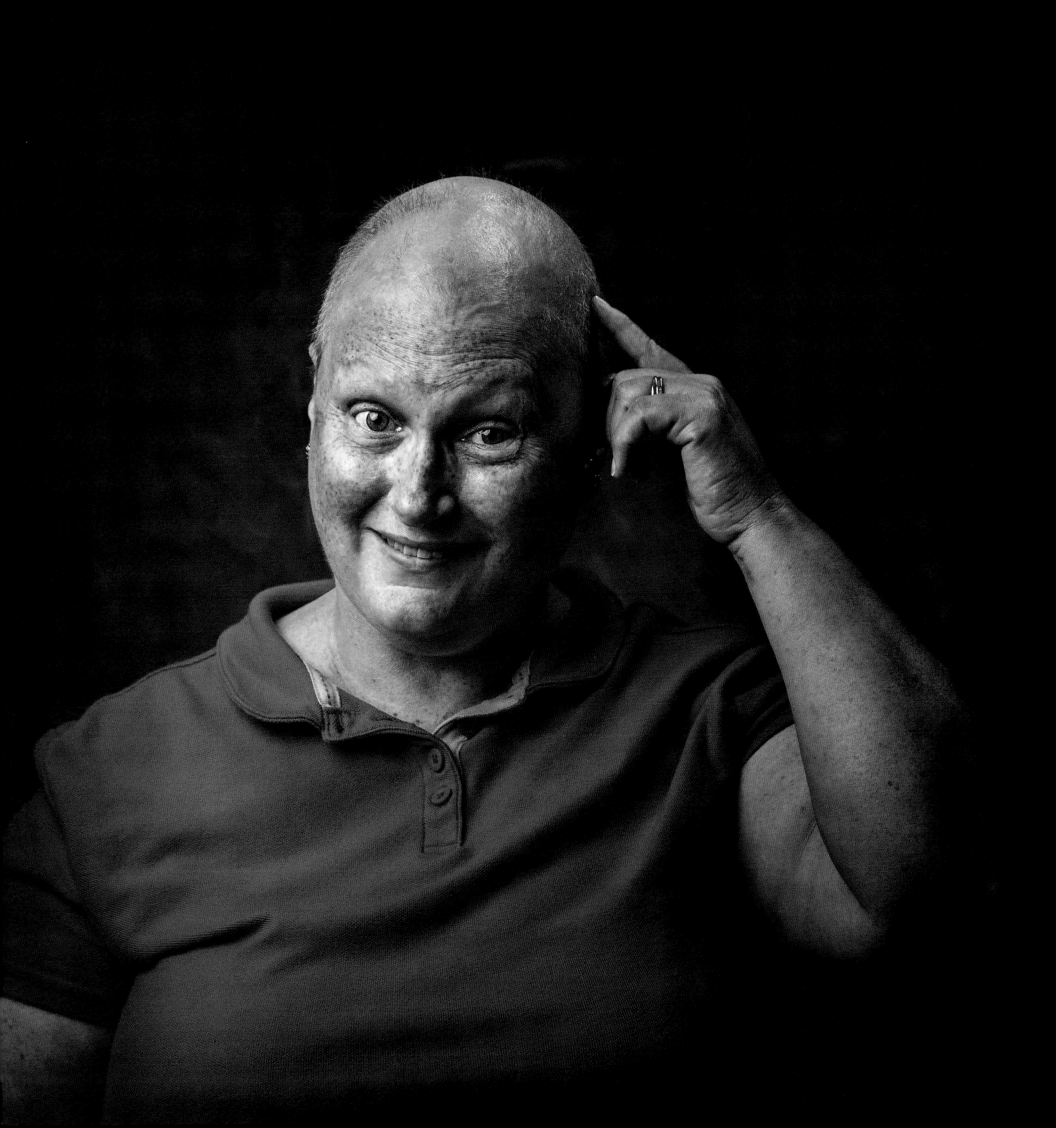

I will, of course, have Herceptin until next July and Zoledronic Acid for three years, but the most unpleasant parts of this journey are over. My hair is growing back but is still very short, so I still wear headscarves most of the time. I was never comfortable in my wig, so I never wore it. Facial hair is coming back with a vengeance! I now have the post-chemo fuzz. If it keeps going, I'd be able to take up a job as Santa Claus at Christmas!

I hope that through this book and my photographs, I can help and inspire, not only photographers, but also those whose lives have been touched by the awful disease we call cancer.

The idea of my body of work called "Faces of Cancer" is to break stereotypical opinions about people with cancer. Everyone dealing with a cancer diagnosis has a different journey, and each journey is as individual as the person undertaking it. Not everyone who has cancer will require chemotherapy or radiotherapy; for a few, surgery alone will suffice, and some people with cancer may not look ill at all. There are so many ups and downs when going through treatment, as people try to cope physically & emotionally with the diagnosis, treatment and side effects. With modern drugs, although chemotherapy causes nausea and vomiting, patients are given a variety of anti-sickness drugs, to prevent them from spending days hunched over a sick bucket, so although nausea does occur, it is now managed far better than in previous years.

Not all drugs cause hair loss, and "cold-capping" which freezes the hair follicles, may slow down or limit the amount of hair that falls out. The side effects of all the drugs affect everyone differently, so every person has a unique story to tell. These images show varying emotions and feelings associated with dealing with a cancer diagnosis and treatment. It features numerous self portraits as well as photos of others, all of whom are either currently undergoing or have had treatment for cancer.

The images are all cropped squarely to create an order in the panel in contrast with the turbulent chaos of cancer. Being in black & white gives a timeless feel to the images, and the gritty, edgy post-production gives a raw and emotional feel to the faces and a sense of truth and reality, very different from many of today's retouched and "perfected" images. The idea is to show the subjects as they are, not as an idealised version of themselves, in order to raise awareness of the emotions, both positive and negative, of cancer sufferers. Several images deliberately break rules in terms of cropping and posing in order to create tension, emotion or discomfort for the viewer.

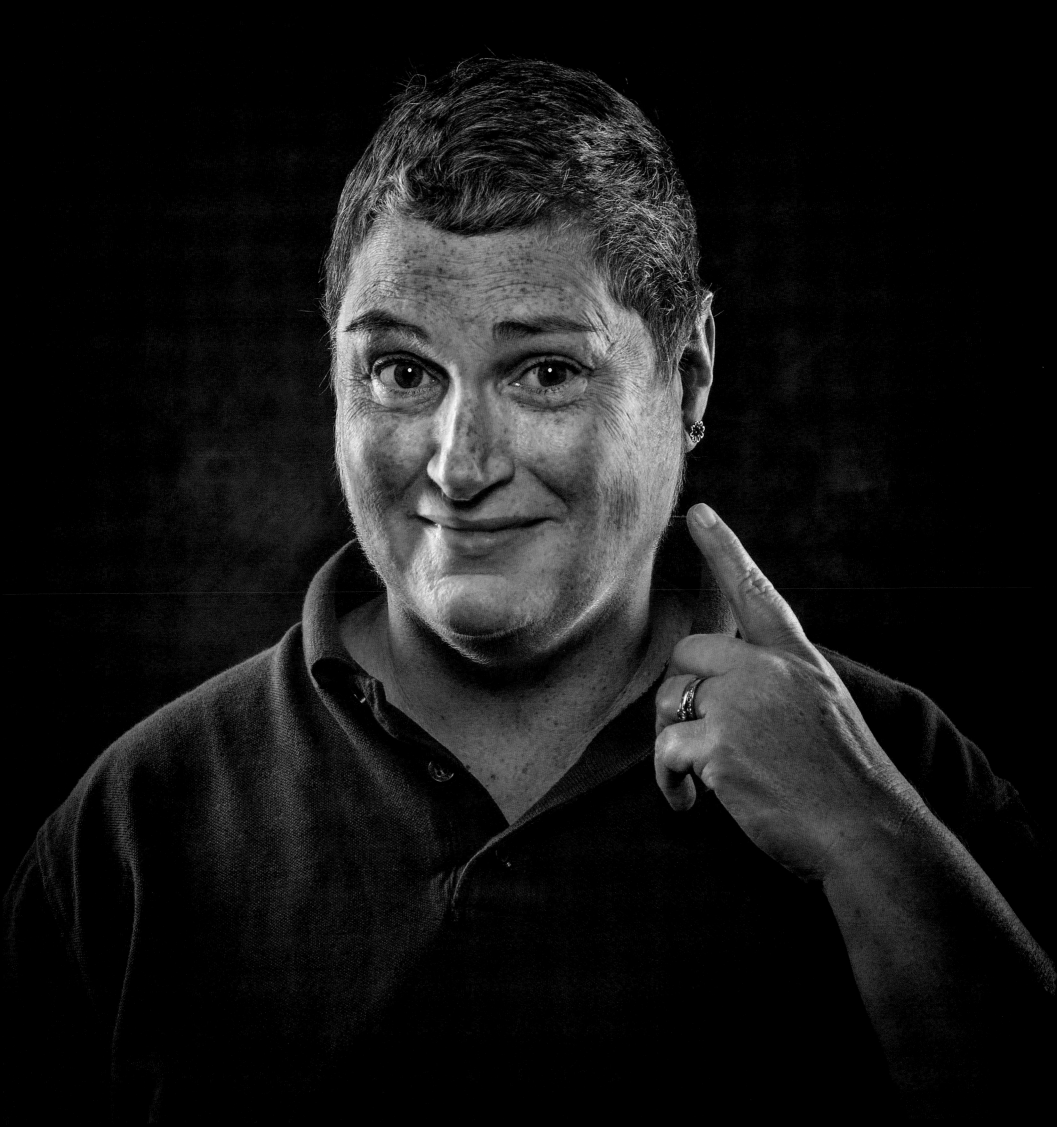

Well....where to start....but......in February I presented at my GP who, thankfully, due to his quick thinking and concern, SAVED MY LIFE! He rushed me into hospital, where within 4 hours, I was told I had a brain tumour and it was suspected to be malignant!!!

I was immediately referred to King's hospital in London and my surgeon advised the tumour would be removed on 7th March (they couldn't be beforehand as there was too much swelling in my brain and yes, they did confirm I have one!!!!)

I remained within Medway Oncology unit for over a week...where I was treated, amazingly I would like to add (as I do know they often receive terrible reports!)

After a few days planned at home, unfortunately I was then taken unwell and rushed up to King's slightly earlier; however the surgery went ahead and due to the wonders of modern technology my tumour, "Paddy" as he was named, was removed, measuring in at a whopping 3.5 x 4 x 4.5cm!

Unfortunately I was then advised that the tumour is a Grade 4 "Glioblastoma multiforme". Basically it is malignant, aggressive and incurable. I was then discharged under the care of the specialist brain tumour team at Maidstone Oncology Centre, whom I met 2 days after my discharge from Kings and I have been under their care ever since. After some time to heal from the surgery, I commenced an intensive period of radiotherapy on 16th April -

every Monday to Friday at the hospital, alongside daily chemotherapy. Unfortunately the chemo was stopped a couple of days early as my blood platelets kept dropping. I was due to have 4 weeks hospital free, but I was then having to go in twice weekly for blood tests, although I think such close monitoring is a good thing and it has continued. I am now awaiting my platelet levels to increase so I can start the next month cycle of chemotherapy.

My prognosis will not be further discussed until the end of this chemo, so it is a waiting game now, literally living day by day!

It goes without saying that my world and that of my closest friends and family has been completely turned around. I am losing my hearing in my right ear; my short-term memory, concentration and thought processes have all been affected, as has my vision and energy levels.

I have had to surrender my driving license and have become completely dependent upon friends and family to support me in so many areas of my life. Those who know me well will completely understand how difficult that has been for "Miss Independent"!

I have been absolutely blown away by all of the support I have received - the visits, messages, shopping trips, lifts etc. just to name the minimum. The support has helped me just as much as all of the drugs have.

Paula

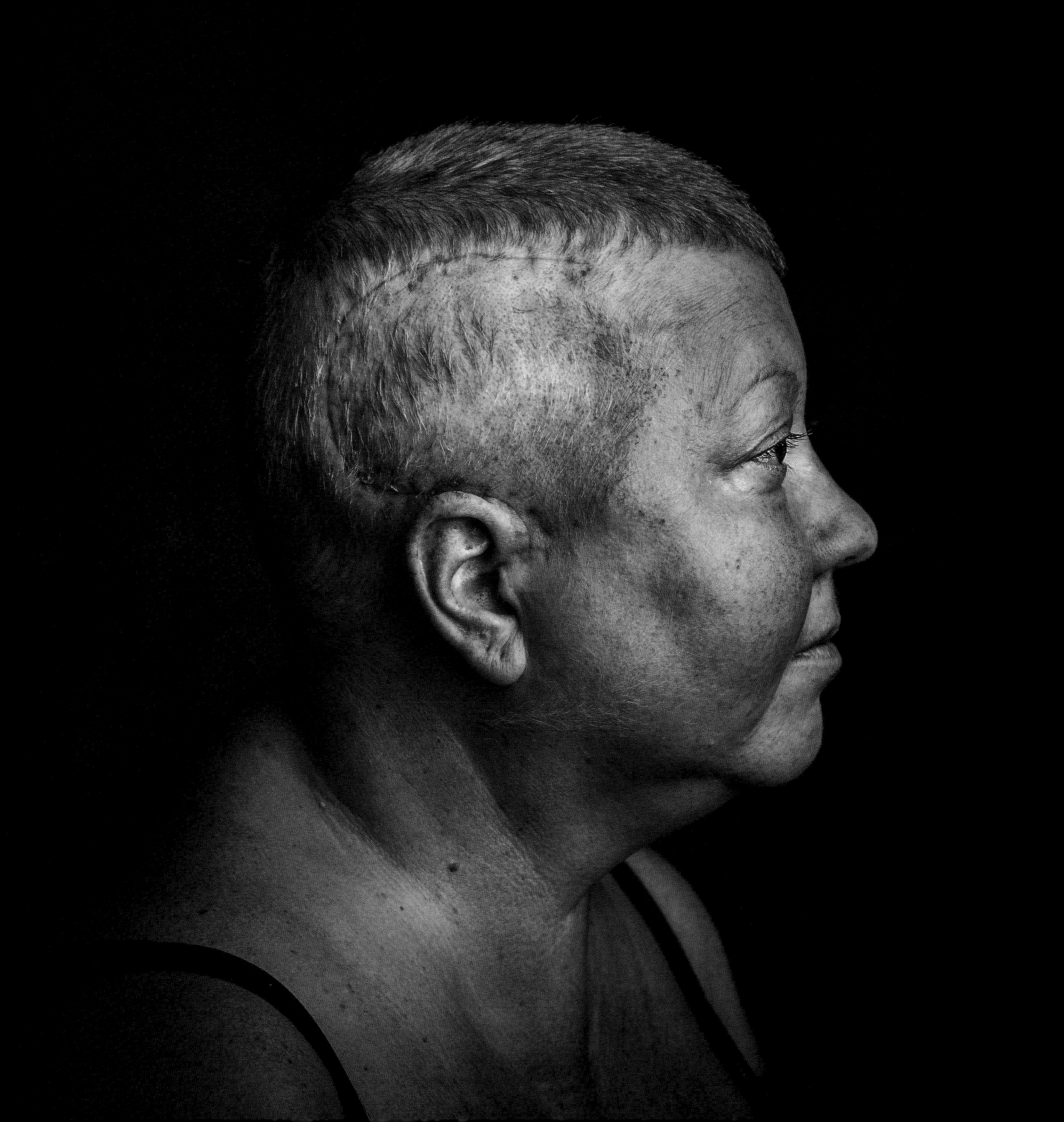

STUART

I was first diagnosed with HER2 positive Breast Cancer in 2005 aged 36 and was really shocked when I was told. I didn't know Men could get Breast Cancer!

When I was told I almost fainted and felt like everything was closing in on me, I started to think about what would happen to my family, my house and was I going to die!

I was in my own bubble for about a week whilst I came to terms with the facts but then I just wanted to get on with everything.

I had a left side Mastectomy and Lymph Node clearance followed by Chemotherapy, Radiotherapy and a new drug at the time called Herceptin. I had to fight to get Herceptin because it was a new drug and my insurance company wouldn't pay for it and my NHS Hospital had no funding to give it to a man with Breast Cancer!

Months of letter writing, radio & TV interviews and a meeting with my MP, Ann Widdecombe, followed. I couldn't have got through it without the help of my wife Karen who wrote to everyone and kept the pressure on the powers that be to get the drug. Eventually an Individual Case Panel sat at my hospital and agreed that I could have it. I remember they called me at work and told me and I broke down after with relief! It felt like a huge weight had been lifted off my shoulders.

I feel that because of all the press coverage at the time it helped raise awareness that Men can get Breast Cancer too.

In 2012 the Cancer returned in my Sternum and I had to have an operation to remove the Sternum at Guys Hospital in London. This was followed by Chemotherapy and another year of Herceptin every three weeks. I was told it was a second primary Breast Cancer, as it appeared so close to the original site.

This second diagnosis was harder for me to take on board mentally but I had great support from my wife and family. I continued to try and stay as positive as possible.

In 2017 I was diagnosed with Secondary Breast Cancer, which had shown up in my lungs. This time I was told that it was treatable but not curable and that I'd have to have Chemotherapy again in conjunction with another two drugs. When the Chemo finished, the two other targeted therapy drugs continued every three weeks and these will continue indefinitely.

I have suffered more with anxiety this time but have been helped a lot by a local charity who have provided counselling, respite breaks and therapies to help me get through it as best as possible. I also have a great group of friends who have had Breast Cancer that I can meet up with and they understand what I'm going through and can help get over any problems or worries.

I have always tried to stay positive and do things to raise awareness of Breast Cancer in Men. Although Cancer is a horrible thing to have it has led to me meeting some incredible people and doing some amazing things which include climbing Ben Nevis, being in two Breast Cancer Care fashion shows as a model and going on a cruise!

I am determined to beat Cancer and stay strong and I think this is portrayed in Imelda's photo of me.

Remember Men get Breast Cancer too.

Stuart

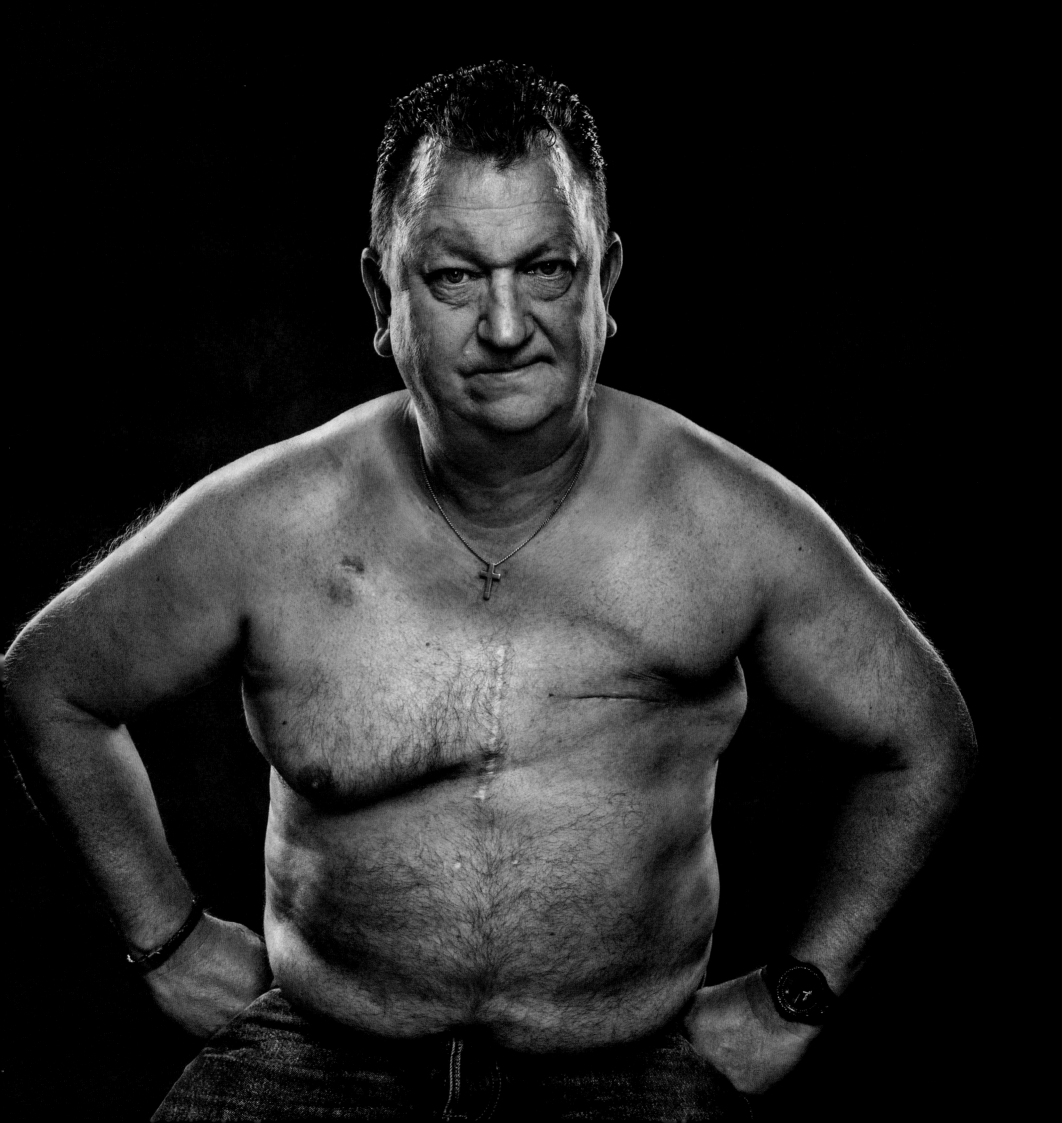

LIZ

It felt as if my life would never be the same again and the future was so uncertain.

Losing my long blond hair was probably my hardest week, which sounds so trivial when you are coping with the brutality of the treatment that is saving your life, but it is about losing your identity, what you think makes you who you are, but when that is taken you soon realise what really matters.

In the love that was shown to me by my friends and family, I have found complete clarity in who was there for me unconditionally, and was and still am overwhelmed by their love and support.

I realise now that not one of us have control over the future, life can change in a nano second; all we have is now, and for me it is about embracing the beautiful relationships that make us who we are.

This is my story .

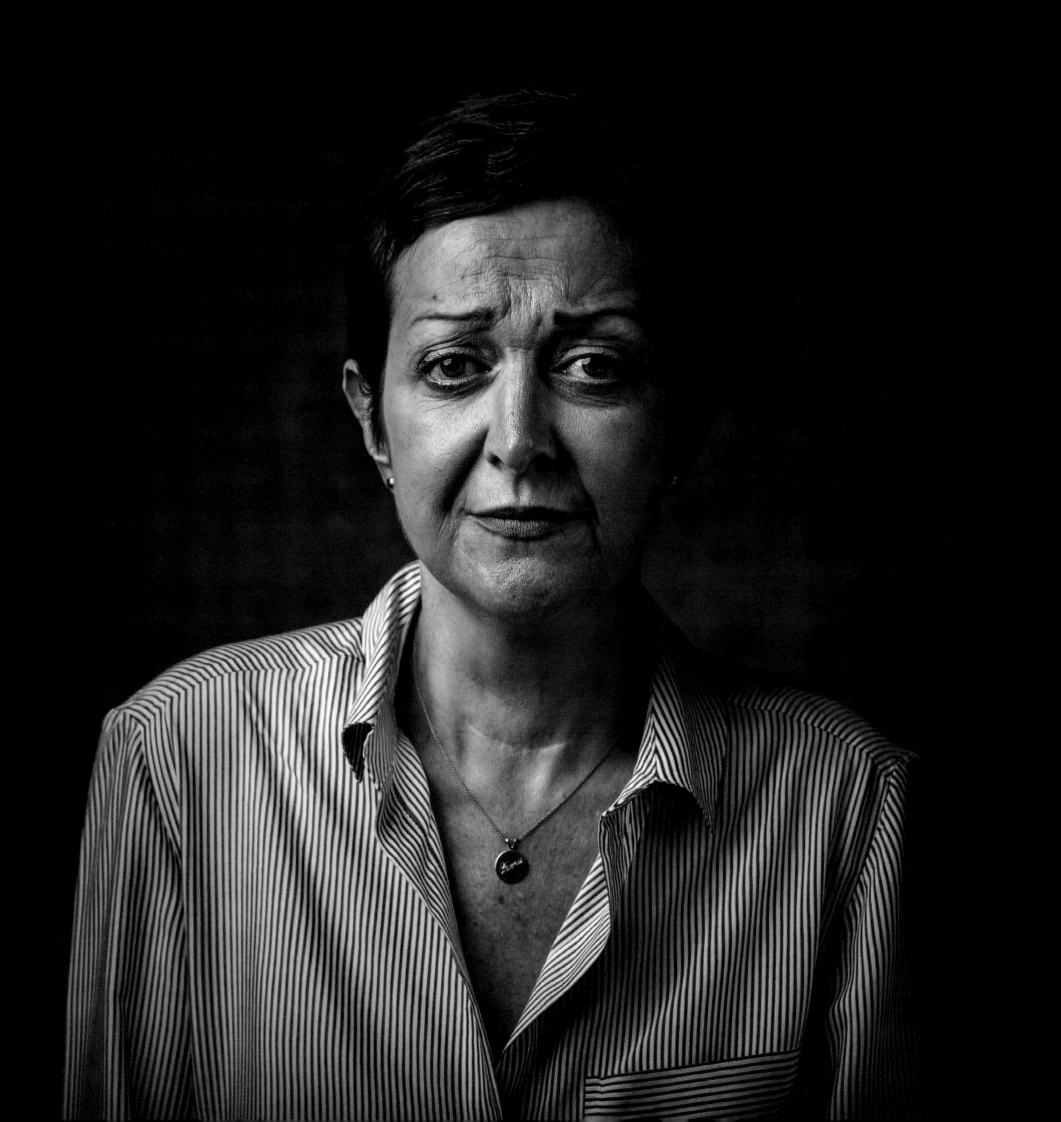

PAUL

I have a grade 4 brain tumour - glioblastoma multiforme.

I was told I didn't have long to live, but I am still alive after four years.

Some days I feel really good, I realise that I am not the only person with problems, there are many people young and old who have a range of problems, I am not alone.

There are other days when I feel really unhappy and think it is pointless carrying on. It is difficult to stop feeling this way, but I do try very hard to be positive.

I am glad I have been alive longer than anyone expected. However, I hate being in limbo, waiting for the regular scan results.

This isn't the life I wanted, but it's the life I've got.

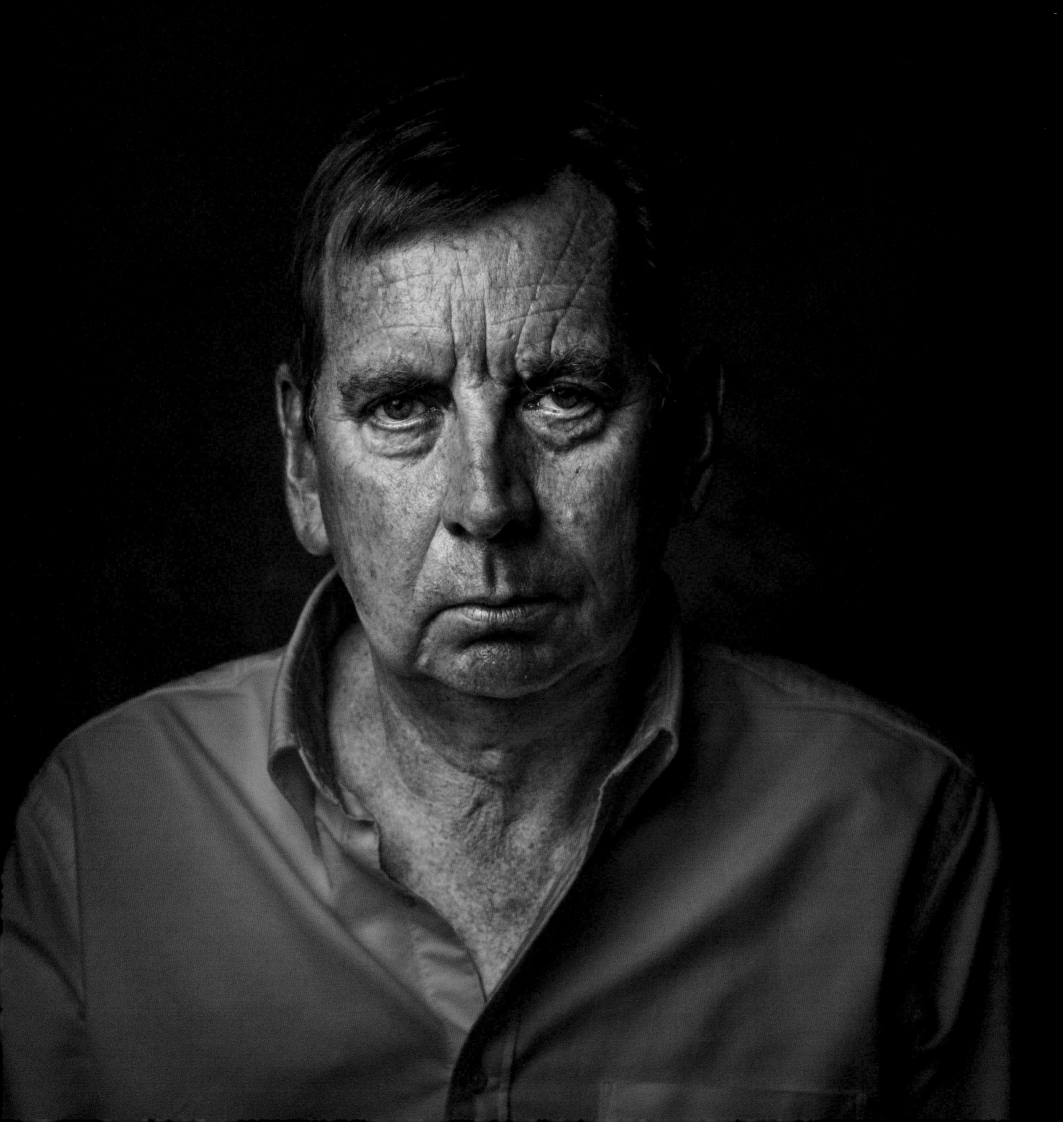

JENNY

I went for my routine mammogram last April in the Tesco car Park. It is never a pleasant experience but it seemed more painful than usual, so I was not that surprised to be called to the hospital for an appointment.

After another mammogram I was told that there was something unusual in my right breast. I then had a scan and biopsies were taken. At this time I felt lucky that I had got to 60 years without any health problems and just hoped that whatever had been found could be removed and I could get on with life.

I then went into another room and met the consultant breast surgeon who explained what would happen next. When we told him that we had medical insurance things moved along at a speed.

The options were explained to my husband and myself and I decided to go for a licap procedure with a reconstruction to be done 3 weeks later. (The lost breast tissue (removed at the time of cancer surgery) is replaced with skin and fat from under your arms). Although I felt scared I knew that Chris, my husband, would support me and we would face all the treatment together.

Surgery went to plan although cancer was found in a node which meant more surgery and chemotherapy as well as radiotherapy.

One of the most difficult things to face was telling our 3 sons and we took each one out by himself to explain what was going on. The second surgery was done and the nodes were removed 3 weeks later, although I found it more painful and took longer to get back on my feet than with the first operation.

August saw the start of chemotherapy, which had its dark times - feeling tired and not able to cook or even eat properly. I didn't want to see anybody and used so much hand sanitizer that I felt I was getting addicted to the stuff! One of the really tough times was when my hair started falling out. I was watching TV, running my fingers through my hair and getting handfuls coming out. I ended up using the hand held hoover to get rid of it. So daft really as I had short-ish, curly hair anyway and I knew it would fall out.

The steroids give you a moon face and the constant runny nose was a nuisance. It really was a case of counting down each chemo and a great achievement when I got halfway through.

My family saw me through it all and my sons coming home each weekend was a great boost as I was still mum even if I was bald!

My wonderful husband turned into a nurse, cook and chauffeur driving me to all the appointments and generally making sure I slept when I came home from the clinic.

I have had wonderful treatment, all the medical staff have been brilliant and I have been very lucky to have so much support and the only time tears came was when we were doing our wills and it all came home to me.

I do think that I have become stronger from having had cancer. As my postman said to me you are now a member of a club that nobody wants to be in.

If I could say anything I would just advise every woman to go to her mammogram appointment, it might save your life, it saved mine.

Jenny

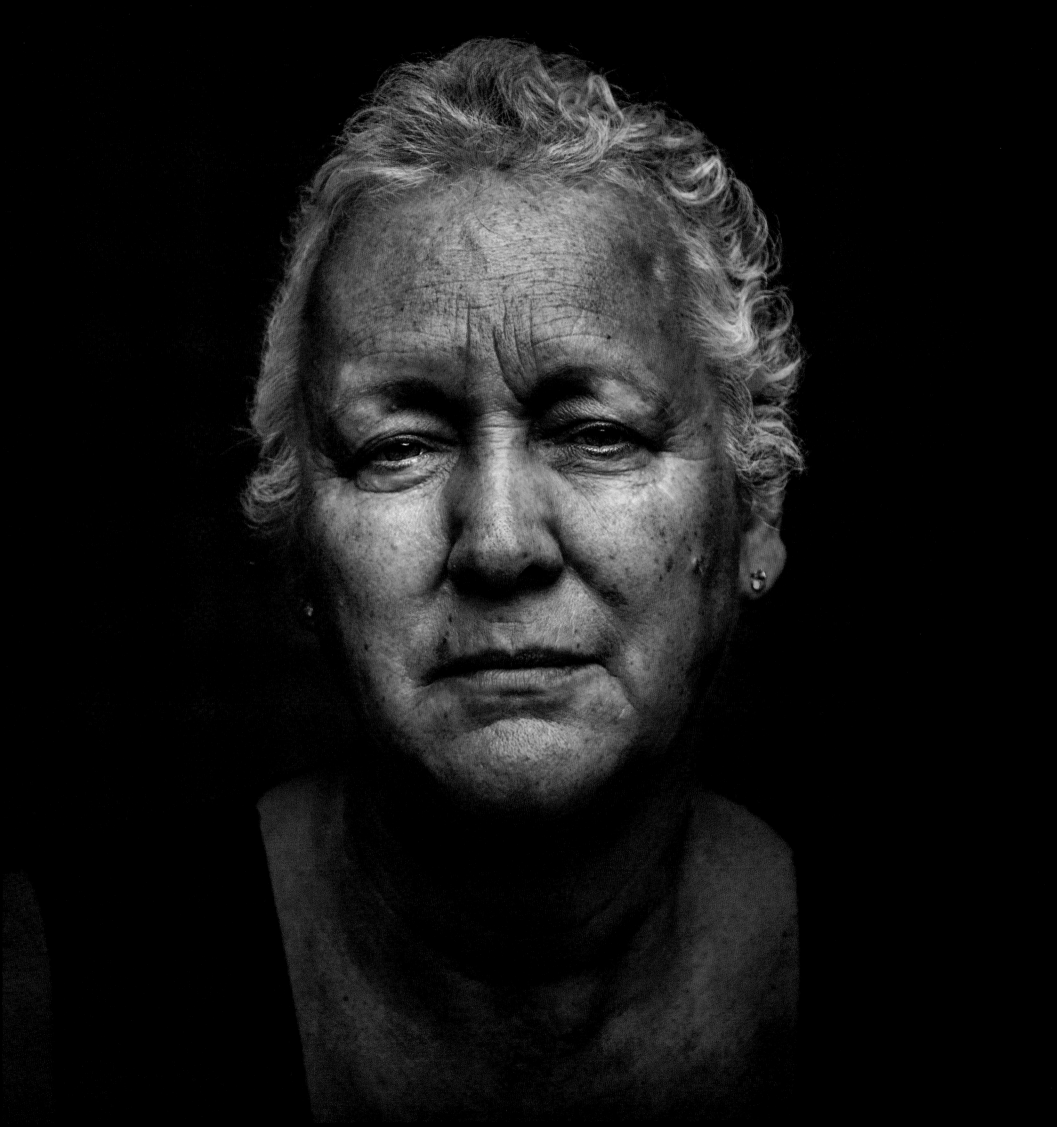

JANE

I never thought that it would be me getting cancer. It was quite ironic though as I was working for two cancer charities at the time I found the lump.

I remember it clearly, standing in the shower. I'm not a great one for checking, but something that day made me think to......

And then the rollercoaster started.

Self detected invasive ductal carcinoma, Chemotherapy, lumpectomy, radiotherapy.

2017 was a pretty awful year for me having to cope with so much not just the diagnosis.

All in all though I consider myself incredibly lucky and blessed and not just because of my family. This diagnosis has given me lots of gifts, resilience, empathy, hope, friendships and a love of life I would not have had previously.

But it is a very lonely place to be, especially when you are awake at 'stupid o'clock' in the morning.

Remember you aren't the only one there are many, many of us out there.

Untitled

The (night) silence is deafening
From the heavy rhythmic pumping of blood in my ears
And the hundreds of questions in my head no one else can hear
And the biggest one....
Will I survive ?
Not just the cancer
Or the chemo
But can I use this to grow?

As a person
As a mum
As me?

The silence is deafening
The anger quite real
Why now at this time?
When I just need to heal

Is this really the universe teaching me how to be?
Or karma finally catching up with me?

Cancer Journey?

It's been described as a 'journey'
A life changing trip!
It feels more like a life sentence
But when do I cash in my chips?!

There are some highs, literally
With the steroids and chemical surges
But the lows are bizarre
With drug induced urges.
This would be so much tougher without you here.

by Jane

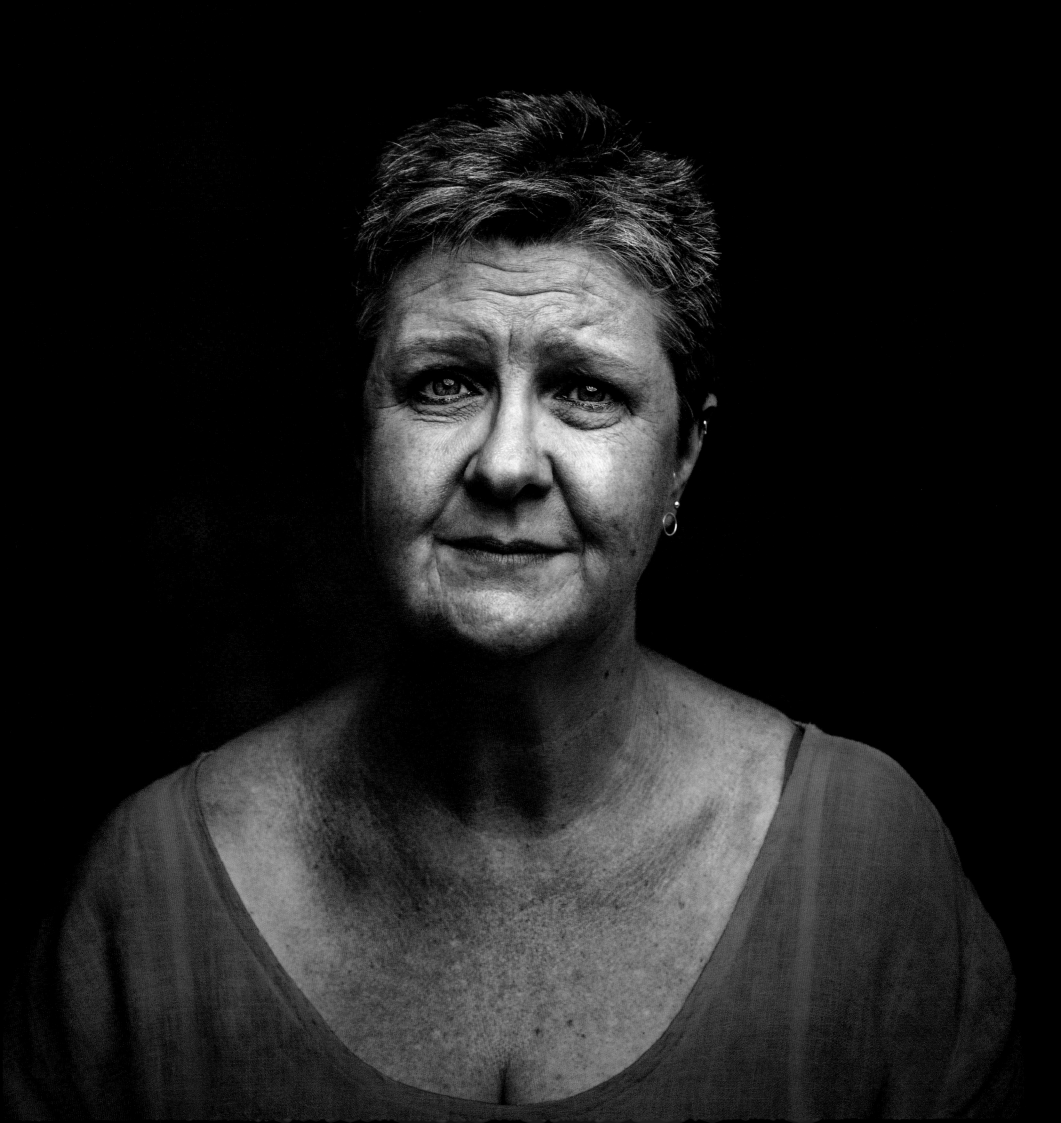

I was first diagnosed with kidney cancer at the end of June 2014 when I was 43. I had my kidney removed, with no requirement for further treatment and spurred on by the enthusiasm of my surgeon and also a friend who had been through the same a year previously, spent the next two years being positively optimistic that it wouldn't come back.

Then it did.

I have advanced Renal Clear Cell Carcinoma in my sternum. I am currently stable and have been for two years. All I need to do is stay alive. There is already a possible cure for my cancer, though it doesn't work for everyone and is not yet generally available. Immunology is at the forefront of current breakthroughs; Jim Allinson and Tasuku Honjo have just been awarded the 2018 Nobel Prize in Medicine for their ground-breaking work.

The second diagnosis was devastating. My oncologist somehow painted the rosiest of pictures, knowing that the immunology work was in the pipeline and I felt positive I could beat it again. I started treatment immediately. Kidney cancer doesn't respond to the chemotherapy that most people associate with cancer treatment. Instead I take my chemo, a biological therapy, orally every day and I'll take it for as long as it continues to work. When it stops working I'll get a new one. It's a challenge mentally because I'm reminded every single day that I have cancer, there's no way to escape it when you have a cocktail of pills to manage – I have pills for pills! The magic cure isn't available to me yet on the NHS, at the stage that I am currently at. I basically need to be on death row – all other options (two of them) used up. If I could be on a trial for earlier stage use of the immunology I would jump at the chance in a heartbeat.

The side effects of my drugs are very similar to traditional chemo and I've been through the gamut of them all. The sickness and diarrhoea have had the nice little bonus of allowing me a brand new wardrobe! I haven't lost my hair, but it's now pure white, as are my eyelashes and eyebrows. Usefully, it's highly fashionable at the moment and apparently it really suits me, though I'm yet to be convinced.

Being out in the sun now creates its own challenges as my melanin production is non-existent and I am the master of cover up. I am permanently cold, probably the only person to carry a cashmere jumper round Florida in July and the Caribbean in October!

Since my second diagnosis I have got married, bought a boat that we hope to sail to the Med next year, changed career, refurbished a house, learned to dive and life is good. I undoubtedly have a different focus. It's an undeniable fact that we get one life, it's beyond precious and I intend to make the very best of it.

I am continuously indebted to my family and friends for their ongoing support and love, which has been entirely unwavering. And to my amazing team at Southend Hospital, who I have the upmost faith in, they're my lifesavers.

Jo

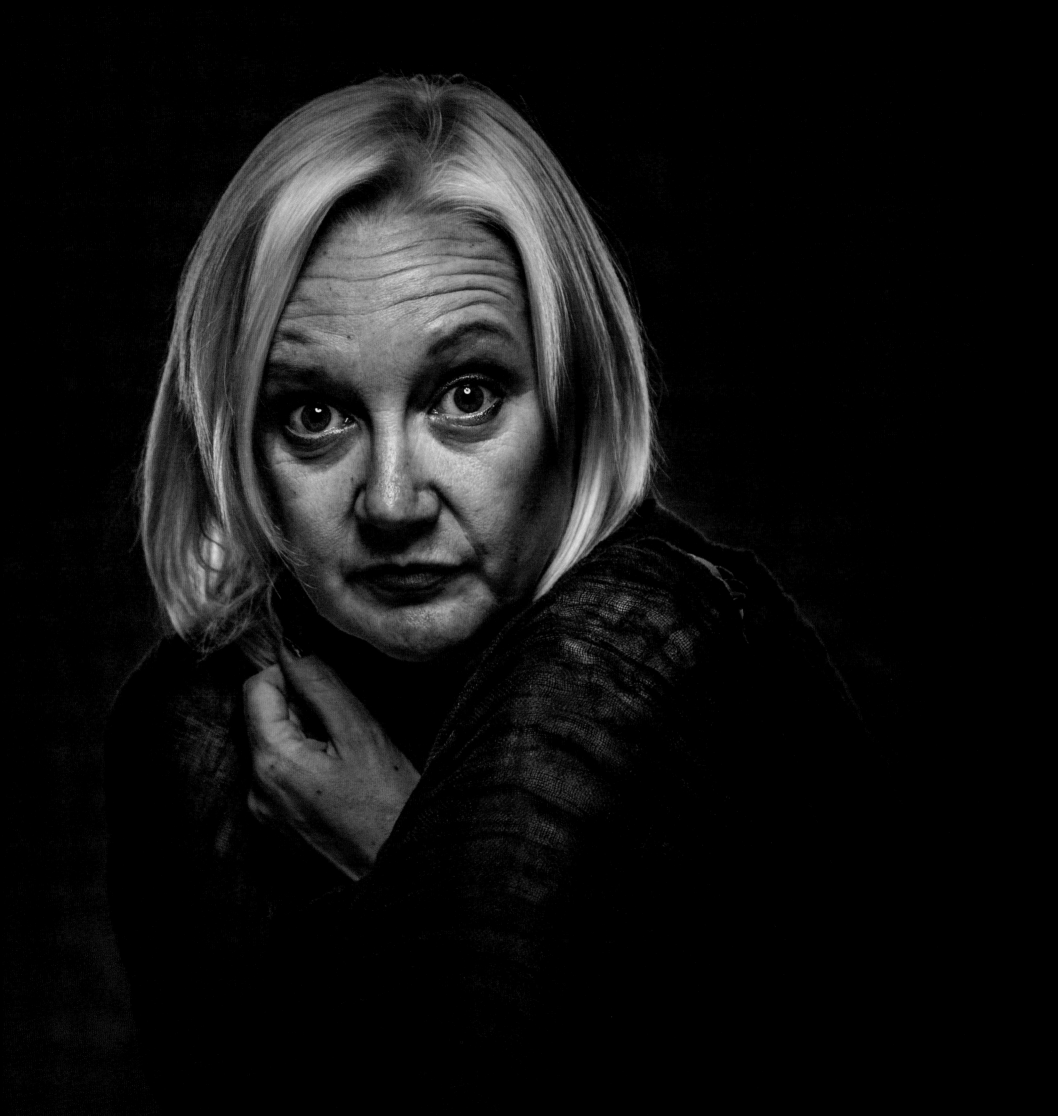

MICHELLE

My name is Michelle and I was adopted as a baby. My mum always said to me growing up that one thing with adopting a baby (back in the late 60s) was that you didn't know the family history relating to illness and hereditary conditions. But we accepted that was that and I trundled through life being an all round good time girl and squeezing every party I could in to my life.

Suddenly one day, my parents received a letter from Guys Hospital and the Church adoption society trying to locate a girl (i.e. me). Two days later I had a counsellor from Guys hospital who told me that my birth mother had died of ovarian cancer (she was in her 40s when she got ill) and all the women had had cancer - I was to be put on a screening programme.

I was 32 years old and devastated! The silver lining was that I had a birth sister - Sarah, who is now my best, best friend! It was hard as I felt like I was just waiting to get cancer, but my scans came back clear each year.

Then in 2016 I felt a sharp pain in my right breast, after a few weeks I plucked up courage and went to my GP who referred me for another mammogram and further tests...the waiting is really the worst part but they knew... I knew and the following week at the age of 48 I developed Stage 3 breast cancer. I was beyond scared, my worst fear had happened - the partying stopped. I had 6 cycles of chemo, surgery and radiotherapy and 17 rounds of Herceptin, which I finished in May 2017. I knew it would be wise for me to have my ovaries out but I just wanted a break from hospitals.

But in February this year I went to the GP as I was bloated and had what I would say were period pains but no period. It was ovarian cancer. Shock and disbelief as well as fear flooded through me again but I was determined to beat it again.

This time I needed surgery first. I had a full hysterectomy as the cancer had spread to my other ovary. I then had 6 rounds of chemo.

This photo was taken after my third round. It was a good day, it was boiling hot and my bald head was sweating uncontrollably but I felt happy!

I set up a blog, which I called Huge Pants to beat Cancer to help get through my dark days and to help others talk about their journey. Cancer is hideous but you do get some gifts. You understand what is important, you understand what love means and you realise who you love and who loves you.

I'm so proud to be a part of Imelda's great Faces of Cancer project - everyone says she captured the essence of me. With or without cancer I'm still a party girl at heart.

Michelle

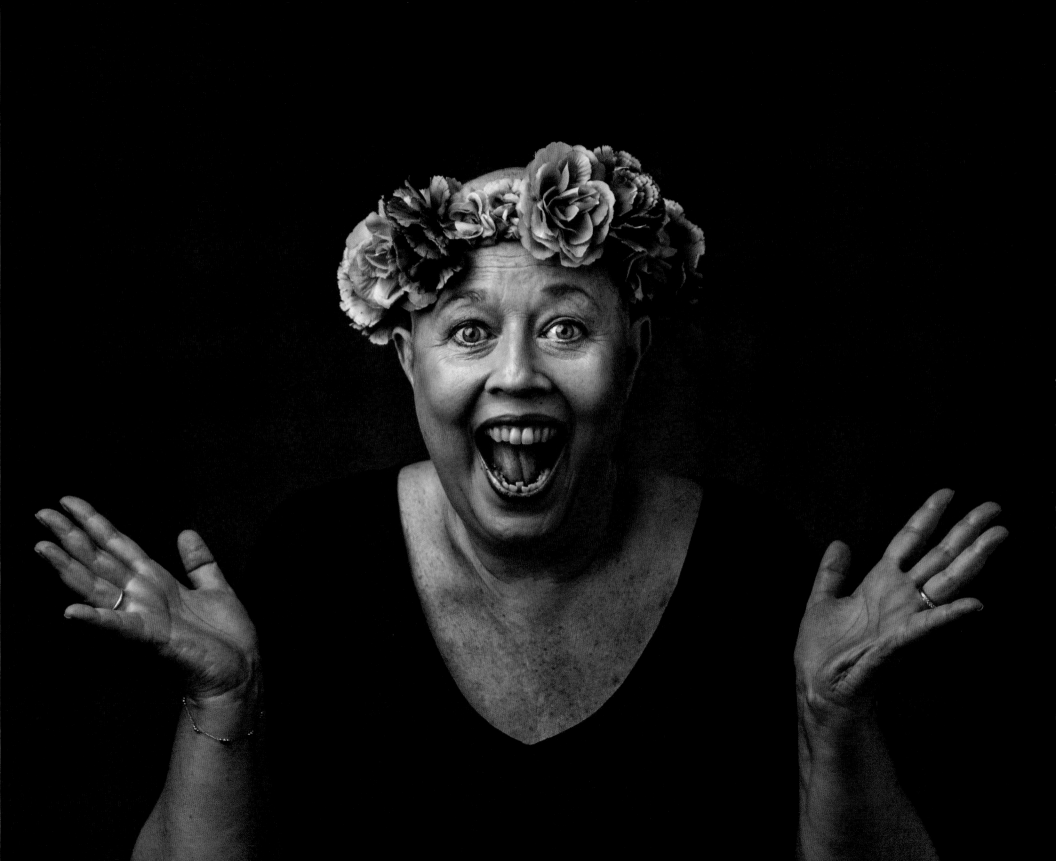

LAUREN

When I found the lump in my left breast back on 16th February 2018, I could not believe it... it was big (4ish cm) and seemed to occupy a large space in the bottom half of my breast. I had never checked my breasts monthly, but did like to think that I didn't completely neglect them! Something in the back of mind propelled me to take my top off and to stand in front of the mirror, with my hands raised above my head; to my horror I saw a 'crater' of a dimple on the underneath of my breast! I knew then that this was trouble... I felt shocked that I hadn't noticed it before now!

Within 4 days, I'd seen a consultant. I went on my own, as naively, I didn't realise I would actually find anything out at that appointment! After a mammogram, ultrasound and biopsy, the consultant told me the large tumour was most probably cancerous, and the biopsy results would confirm what type. I remember sitting there just repeating "okay" in response to everything he told me, feeling quite numb.

A week later he delivered the news that I had a grade 3 invasive ductal carcinoma and was HER2 positive. It all felt so surreal – where in the world had this come from?? I care full-time for my disabled mother and have two children aged 13 and 10. I'm used to being the rock in my family, and could not believe that this was actually happening to ME.

For the next two weeks I felt like I was in a whirlwind and I had a myriad of appointments at 4 different hospitals. My oncologist explained that the best chance I had was to have neo-adjuvant chemotherapy with two targeted therapy (biological) drugs (a delightful cocktail known as TCHP) and then have surgery and radiotherapy after. This truly scared the whatsit out of me, as all I wanted was to have it cut out of me ASAP!!

On 13th March, the 'fun' treatment began! I remember the nurse giving me print outs of all the drugs I was having and the lists of side effects were horrendous. I'd always been the 'Queen of Google' but made the decision there and then to knock that on the head! I was to have 6 cycles, every 3 weeks, and then continue having Herceptin on its own for a further 12 cycles.

Chemotherapy is different for everyone, but general consensus is that it's the PITS! It affects you physically and mentally. Aside from the hair loss, sickness and horrendous diarrhoea, one of the worst things for me was the feeling of just not knowing what to do with myself. I was trying to stay positive for me and my family, but there were times where I felt so low, and really struggled to cope with it all.

And then something AMAZING happened!! My breast nurse convinced me to go along to a Macmillan coffee morning... Going to that meeting, was without a doubt the best decision I've made this year! I was able to laugh and talk to people that really understood what I was going through, and they could give me great advice. You can have the best supportive friends & family in the world, but if they haven't been through this process, they simply cannot understand what it does to you. I now attend these meetings every month, and have made some FABULOUS new friends.

I had my first surgery at the end of July, three weeks after finishing chemo- a lumpectomy and sentinel node biopsy, which basically reduced my breast to around half the size of the other one. This has amused my children no end and given me the nicknames "Miss Odd-titty" and "Little Miss Pert One". Fortunately I do have a FANTASTIC sense of humour! ☺

Four weeks of radiotherapy followed this, which was honestly ok, just tiring going EVERY week day! I had to use the DIBH (Deep Inspiration Breath Hold) technique to lift my chest away from my heart, but the radiotherapy team were great at helping me relax.

It's been a mad 8 months; a complete rollercoaster of a ride and my world has been tipped upside down. I've learnt a lot along the way, particularly how strong you can be when you have to, but also, it's ok to be selfish and put yourself first...Oh and things NOT to say to someone with cancer... e.g. "Sorry I haven't called you for 6 months – I didn't know what to say...."

Lauren

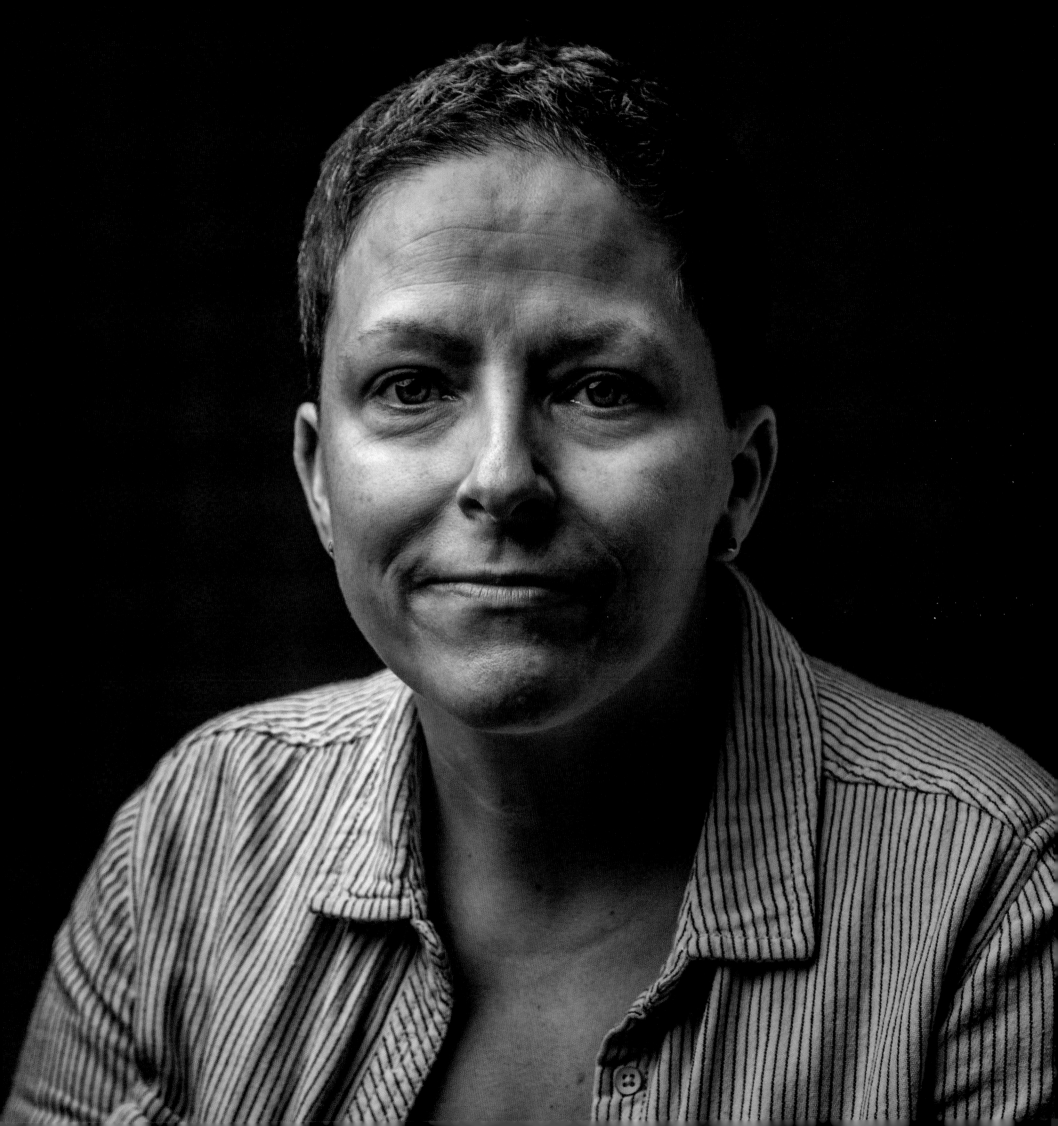

DONIA

On April 21st, 2017, I got diagnosed with three very large tumours in my breast, which had spread to my lymph nodes. At the time I was still breastfeeding my youngest child so didn't in a million years expect to have breast cancer considering I never drank, smoked and lived a healthy life so the moment the Doctor said the words 'You have Cancer' I felt an immediate death sentence was on the cards and my whole world felt like it had just crumbled in front of me.

The next week I grieved every day, every moment I would break down in tears. 'Cancer' I can't have cancer I'm too young to have cancer. I've got two babies who need me this can't be happening to me. I became all-practical and organised all the financial side of things in preparation for my death. I even contemplated vetting a new stepmother for my children. The thoughts which were going around in my head were unexplainable.

Within the last year I don't know how I've managed but amongst the trillion hospital appointments, I've learnt how to self-inject and I'm terrified of needles!18 rounds of chemo, 8x A&E admissions, 4 Ambulance call outs, 16x courses of Intravenous and oral antibiotics, a concoction of daily medication, collapsed veins, chronic bone pain, neuropathy, blood transfusion, blood clot in arm, anaphylactic shock and numerous infections including Sepsis. On top of that I have been brought into early menopause and half way through treatment got confirmed with the BRCA2 gene and I had to have a double mastectomy & a lymph node clearance operation and I also I had to have my fallopian tubes and ovaries removed to reduce my risk of Ovarian Cancer as I am at high risk.

After my initial diagnosis had sunk in, I decided there was no point worrying about something I had no control over, so I decided to take the control over my happiness instead and live each day the best I could. I decided to keep my career as Managing Director of internationally renowned children's modelling and acting agency, Tiny Angels, and try and live my life as normal as possible.

I then found inner strength and decided I wanted to write a book to help my family and other parents cope with explaining a cancer diagnosis to their children.

I have been fortunate to have had the wonderful Joanna Lumley on board who wrote a lovely quote on the back of the cover for me. I have various charities on board supporting this book where I will be donating some of the proceeds of the book and the charities are the Royal Marsden charity which is where I am currently undergoing treatment still, Cancer Active Charity, the willow foundation charity, Taylor Made dreams charity and the look good feel good cancer charity.

On an even more exciting note, I am working with a film producer and script writer who are currently turning my first book of the series into a feature film.

I never in a million years thought all these wonderful things would happen from something so traumatic but where there is hope there is life. I was told I only had a 60% survival in the first year but I fought with every bone in my body as I was not giving up!

Life is so very precious, I hope you find some inspiration from my journey to keep going no matter what life throws at you.

Donia

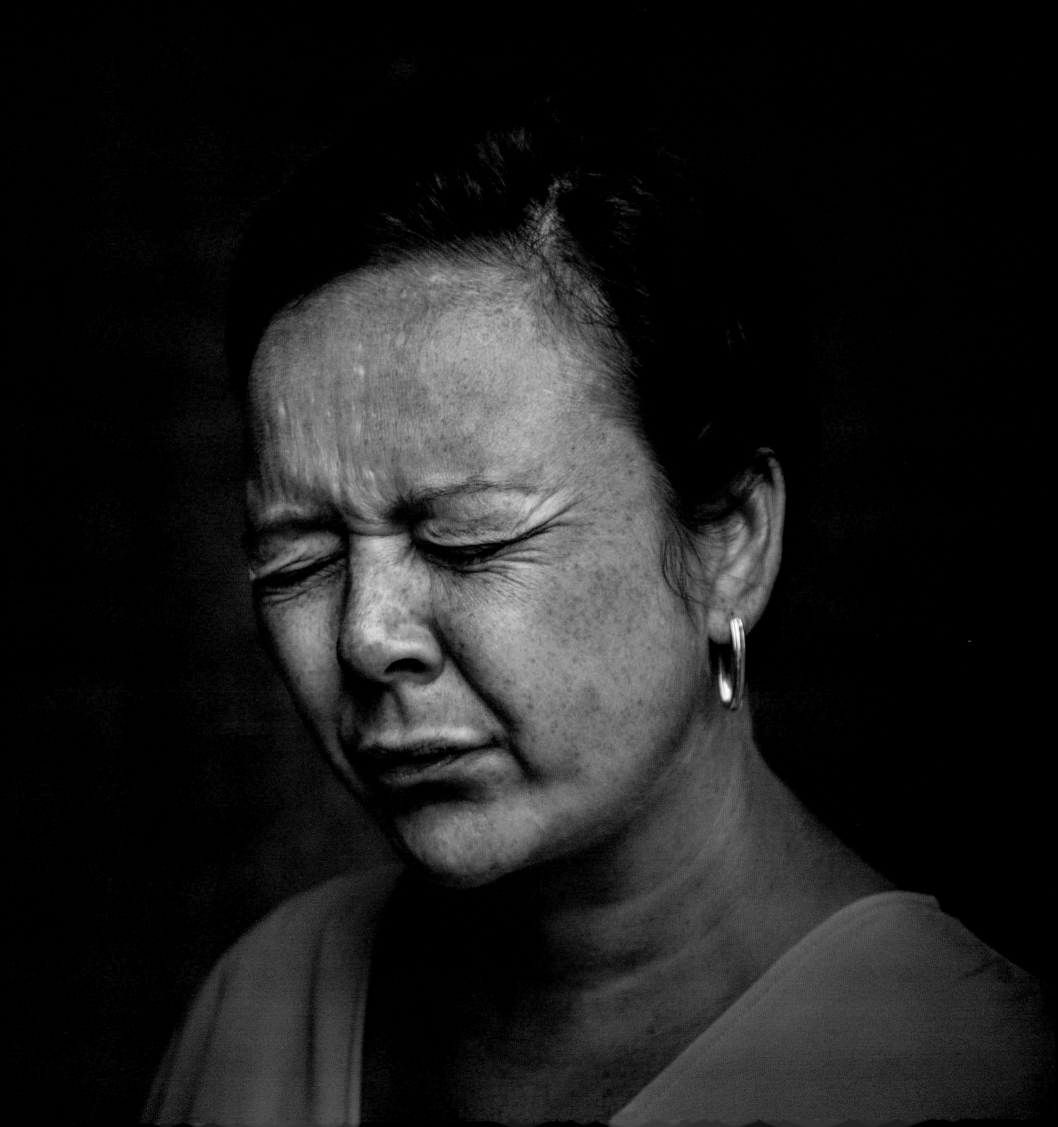

EMMA

I was diagnosed with invasive lobular breast cancer in October 2017.

I had a mastectomy, chemotherapy and 15 radiotherapy sessions in the space of 10 months. I decided to tackle my tumour - which was 95mm - with humour. From the start I found myself making jokes and laughing at the situation I was in. It was my way of coping. I had initially been fairly ignorant of what was going to lie ahead of me. Then one night I made the big mistake of searching for answers on the internet. I frightened myself and was convinced I was going to die. I decluttered the house, made a will, and wrapped Christmas presents early in case I didn't make it! Chemotherapy was worse than I thought it would be. I didn't mind losing my hair but losing my taste buds was awful. Water was revolting; tea tasted like metal and chocolate seemed to sting in the mouth. I couldn't watch TV or read and sleeping made me feel worse. The dizzy spells and pain was at times intolerable. The first week of each chemo cycle was the worst, but I kept my sense of humour throughout and recorded my journey. I even dressed up as bald celebrities and produced a comedy charity calendar for Breast Cancer Care. I started an Instagram page and took great comfort laughing and joking with others going through similar treatment. I miss my bald head but I am so thankful I have got this far, knowing others have not been so fortunate. The cancer has made me stronger, wiser and actually happier as I have realised exactly what is important in my life.

Emma

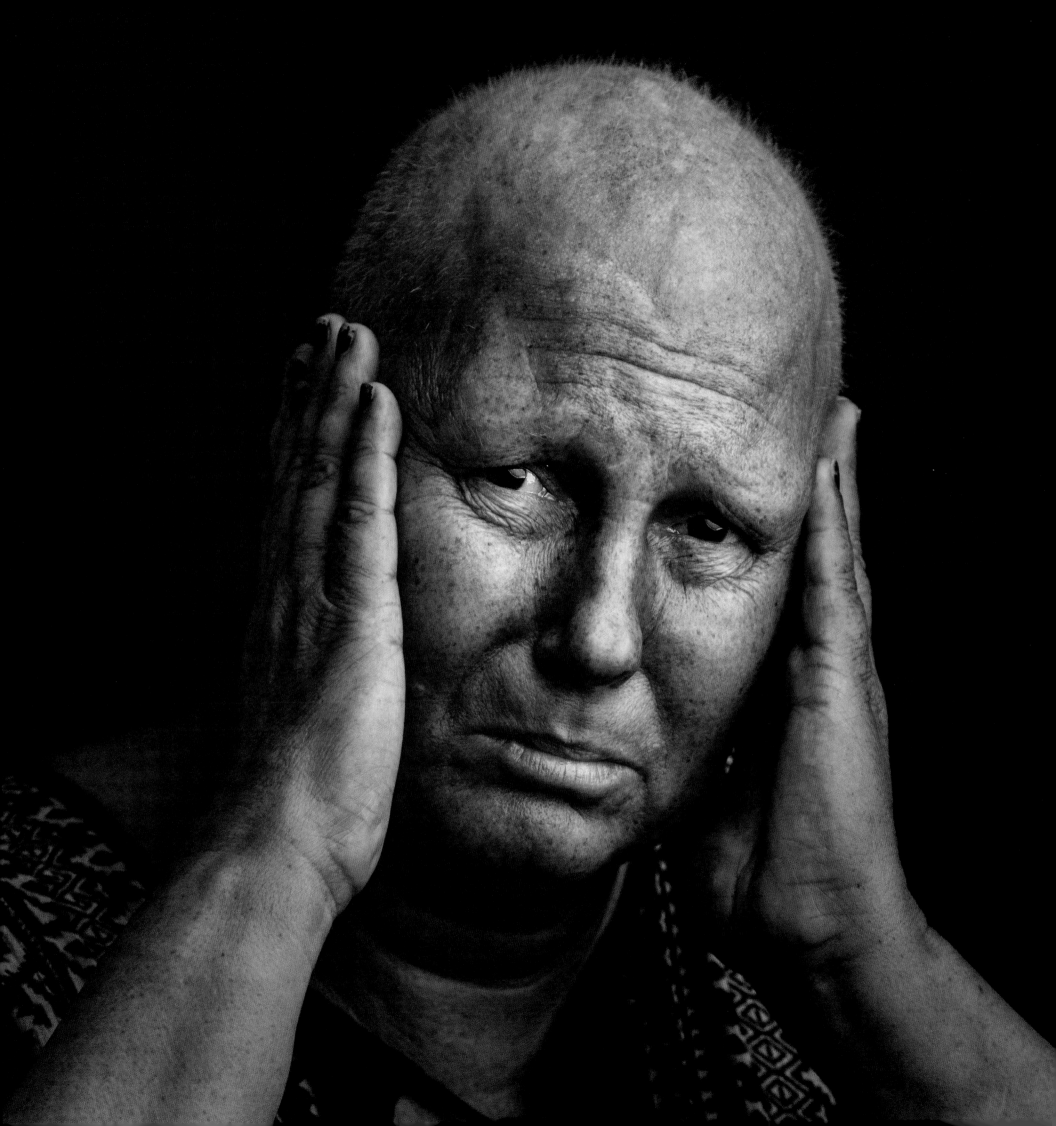

BRUCE

I was diagnosed with Oesophageal Cancer in May 2014 after a lengthy period of knowing I was ill, but failing to convince my GP.

My prognosis was not great (common with this cancer). This made it a completely life changing announcement.

I never thought about my death and what it would be. Now it dominated everything. My every waking thought and my dreams were dominated by my demise.

I was offered surgery to remove my oesophagus and 75% of my stomach. This would come with both pre & post operative Chemotherapy. I agreed to this and by December 2014 I was home and starting my recovery.

My cancer changed me. The realisation of my failings as a father and a husband hit me hard. I guess, I always thought I would fix these things. Now I didn't have the time or the strength.

Now I needed my family so much. The family that I had, so many times just taken for granted. I love them so much, the words would not come. But it did and it has. But I know I will never live up too the role that I took on as a father and husband.

Sadly for us all my cancer has returned. I have now undergone further Radiotherapy but have declined Chemo in favour of quality of life. What I have left I want to give to my family.

To anybody out there reading this. Hug your family now, tell them you love them now. Show you mean it now. You may not get tomorrow to do that.

Bruce

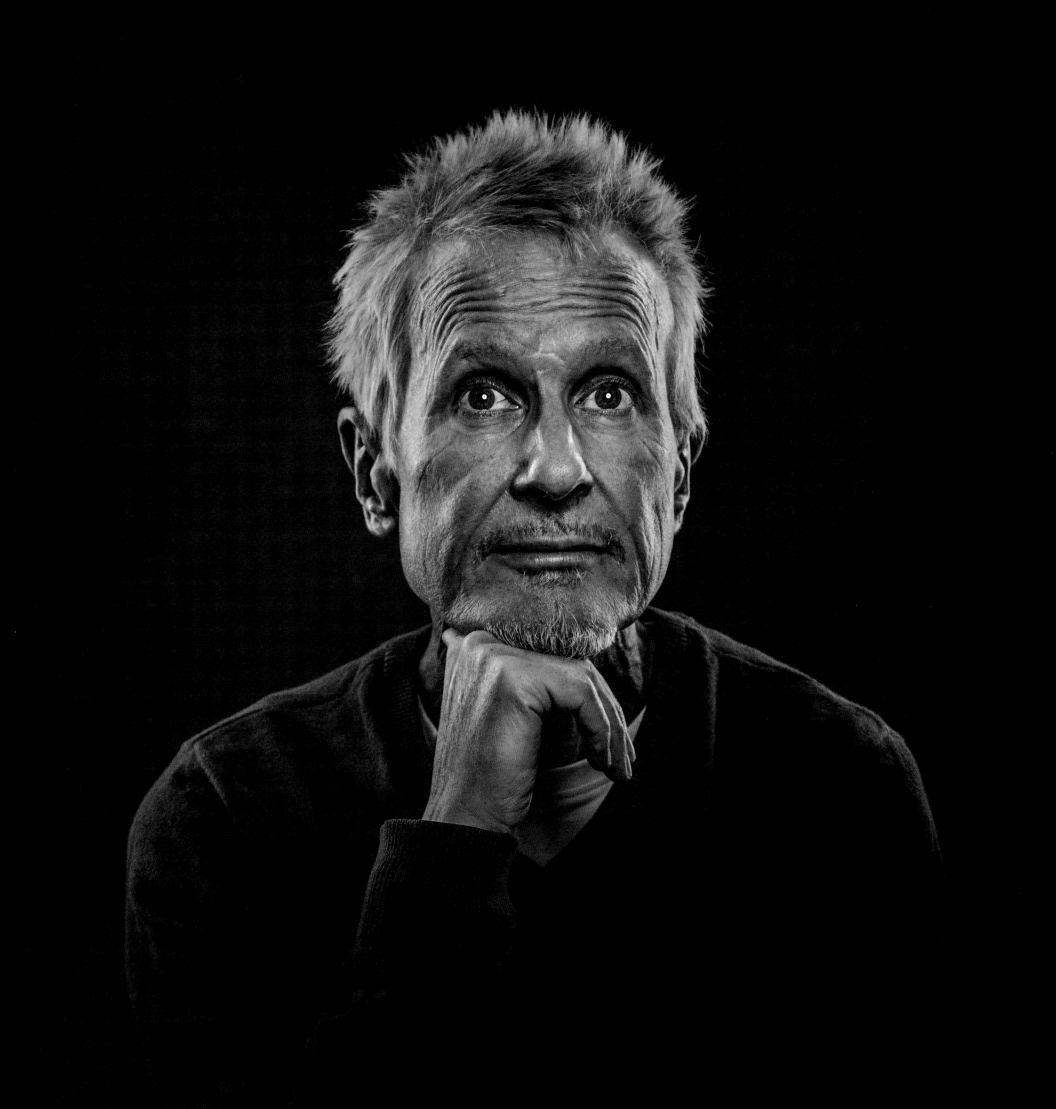

LISA

To hear I have cancer at thirty five,
I sit and wonder how long will I be alive,
months of chemo and losing all my hair,
feeling like all people do is stare.

A mouth full of ulcers, no food tastes the same,
I certainly needed to up my chilli game!
Lots of time alone in my bed,
with all sorts of thoughts going through my head.

Never have I been so lonely watching the world
carry on,
so much I want to do but my journey is so long,
people come to visit and feel me with cheer,
when they leave again I shed a tear.

No one gets how cancer makes me feel,
it's like my life has paused standing still,
I miss lots of parties and having fun,
see lots off photos but I'm in none.

I sit and I wonder when this will end,
wearing a fake smile I often pretend.
End of chemo day comes, a big part is done,
my hair will start growing , when will I have a bun?

People then say "that's it, you're done!"
if only they knew the mental journey has just
begun.
I may look better but inside I'm broken,
strange ,horrid thoughts none of it spoken.

I start to talk and open up, now things seem ok,
I've got this, today's a good day.
Then to be told you have beat the big C,
look at my face this is me.
happy , excited ,very grateful to be .....
CANCER FREE!!!!

Lisa

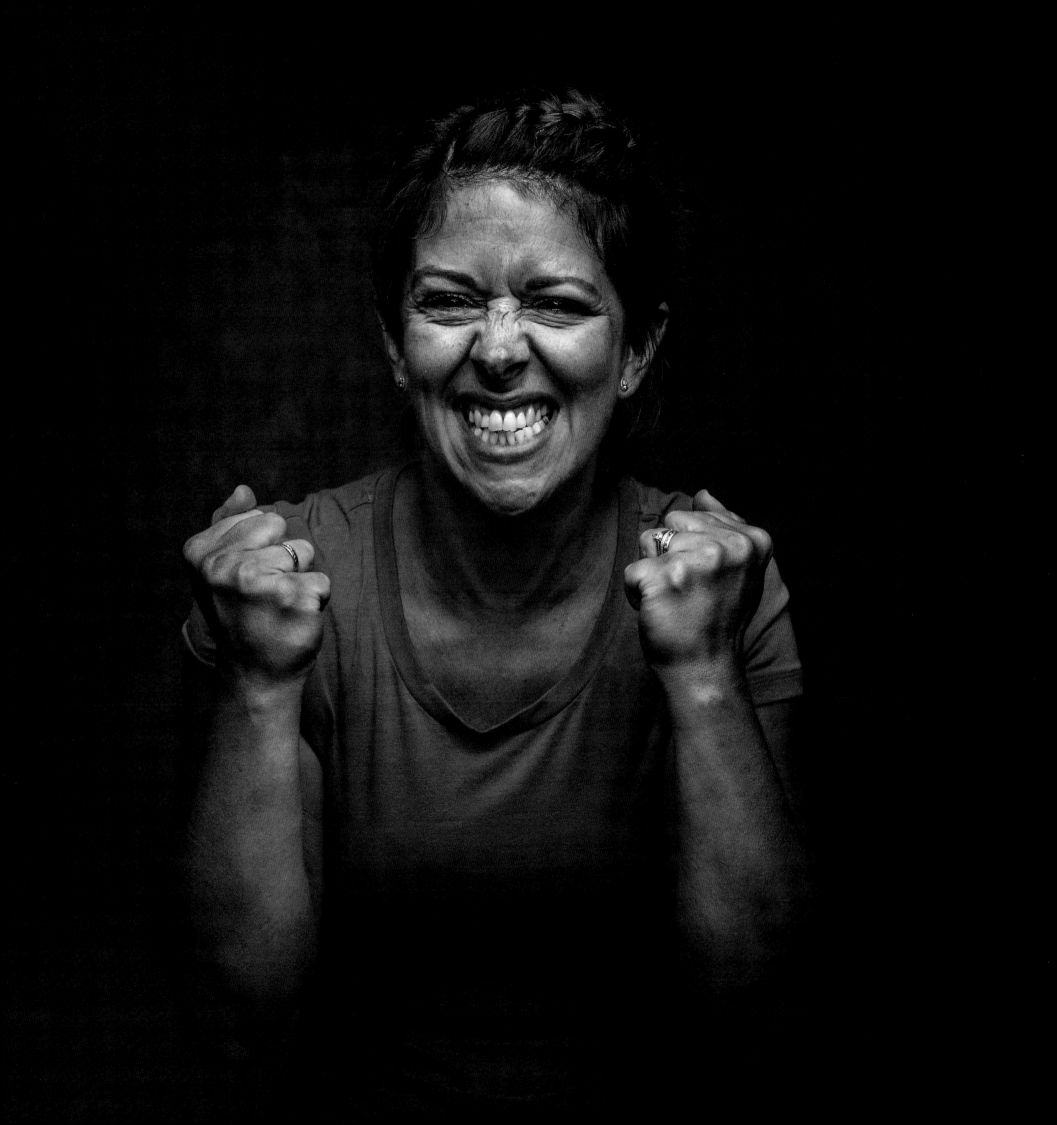

CARA

I never really liked my breasts
They hung and swung and hurt
They were 32GG
They nearly reached my skirt!

So off I went to have them shrunk
'You'll have to have a scan...
There might be something in there
So we'll catch it if we can '

Low and behold, the scan it showed
A thing called DCIS
It was early but spread far and wide
So I'd lose it nonetheless

The right one was the problem
The left one was okay
I thought and made my mind up
They would both be on their way

I couldn't live with one large breast
All heavy there and swaying
Whilst on the right there'd be a scar
That's not a game I'm playing...

The surgeon didn't like that much
'You'll have to go elsewhere
To get a second opinion
See...we think it's only fair '

It's my body though is it not?
My choice my life, my right?
'You can't have both removed my dear...
Well, not without a fight

'I'll do it but you realise it's
What makes you feminine....'
Oh that's okay I say
It's a fight I have to win

So now I'm flat and firm and free of cancer
So that's great
My husband did a runner
Turns out he wasn't my best mate

People think I'm odd you know
To not want some fake mounds
But I just don't see the point
More surgery is out of bounds

So life and me look different now
Some clothes they just don't fit
But hey I'm here and living life
And dealing with this shit!

Cara

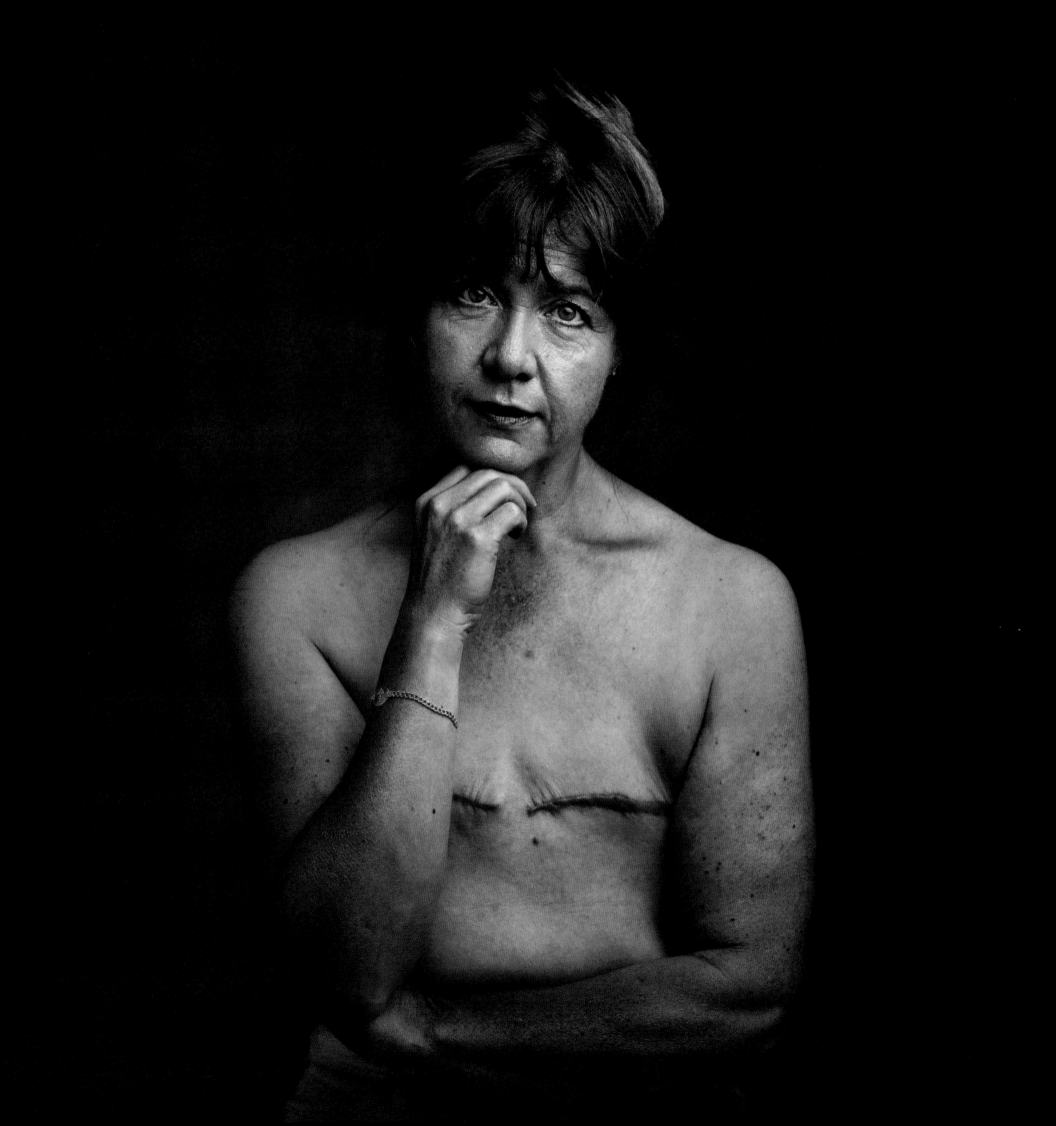

LUKE

My story started 2 days after my 17th birthday.

I had to go to the hospital to collect my biopsy results. I didn't really understand what a biopsy was for, I just thought they would tell me I had a viral infection and give me some antibiotics. Instead, they told me I needed to start chemotherapy. My heart sank and I freaked out, I was so scared of losing my hair and I was terrified of the fact that my brothers and sisters could lose me. I didn't know how I was going to tell them, I couldn't tell them, I just apologised repeatedly.

After a few days I accepted the fact I was ill and I was ready to fight. I remember lying in the hospital bed whilst waiting for the results, I thought it was only stage 1 as it was only my neck that was hurting, but I remember waking up and hearing the doctor say it was stage 4 and it was everywhere, I was smothered with it.

Because the cancer was so severe I had to have two different types of chemo. The first time I had both lots of chemo it made me very ill, but I got over it quickly and recovered.

The great thing is that the chemo completely destroyed all the cancer cells and after 2 to 3 cycles I was in remission, I had won the battle!

I've always said to people that have asked, the chemo isn't that bad once you're used to it, the hardest thing for me was being so far away from my family and not seeing them for long periods of time.

But cancer is not all bad, there is good that comes from it, you make new lifelong friends, and you realise who is really there for you. You become closer with your family and you learn a lot of life lessons.

Never take anything for granted cause it can be taken away so quickly, I've learnt to appreciate everything I have in my life. So although cancer is a horrible disease, a lot of good comes from it too.

Luke

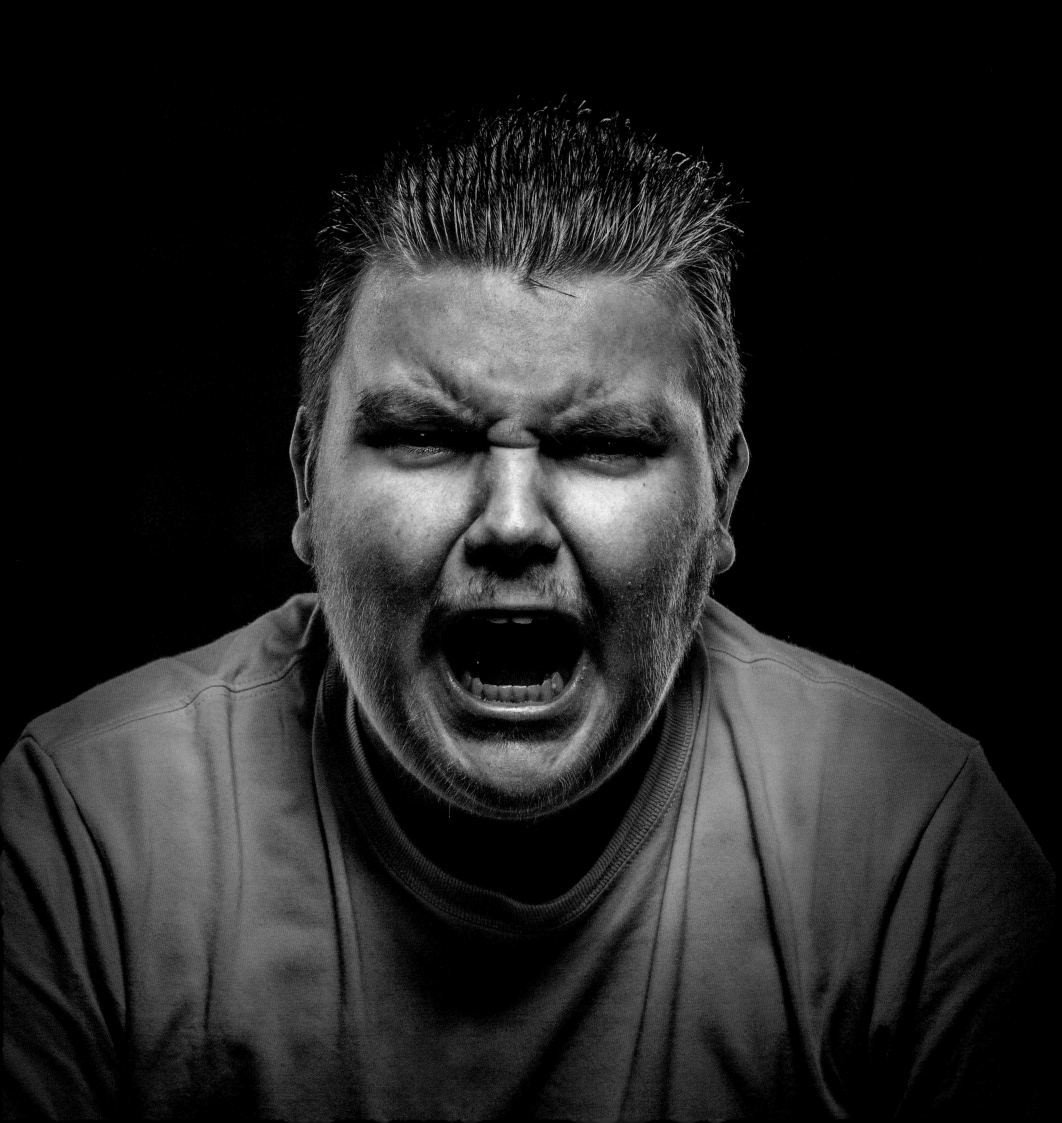

MICHELE

All I can say is survivor of Grade 3 Cancer
And still fighting the fight.

Diagnosis

I hear the words, "It's cancer"
My mind goes blank.
I can't speak, I can't think.
I am dazed and numbed
By the discord of my emotions.

Fear creeps into my soul and grasps my heart
With an icy hand and a vice like grip.
Dread climbs from my toes
Clawing at my sinews until it reaches the tip of my head
Where it explodes in a frigid torrent of terror.

Sweat trickles down between my shoulder blades
And puddles in the small of my back
My breath restricts as panic rises from

The deep pit of my churning stomach
And a moan ascends from the boiling maelstrom below.

My head buzzes as thoughts rub together
in a frenzied dance
to the hum drum of my heartbeat
and the whoosh of the blood pounding my ears.

My knees start to tremble and buckle
And I stand outside my body
Detached and severed
Looking in at the turbulent furor
Which threatens to engulf my existence.

I want to shout, I want to run
But I am rooted to the spot
Cold and paralysed
Stuck at this juncture with the heinous cackle
Of this vile disease echoing in my every thought.

by Imelda Bell

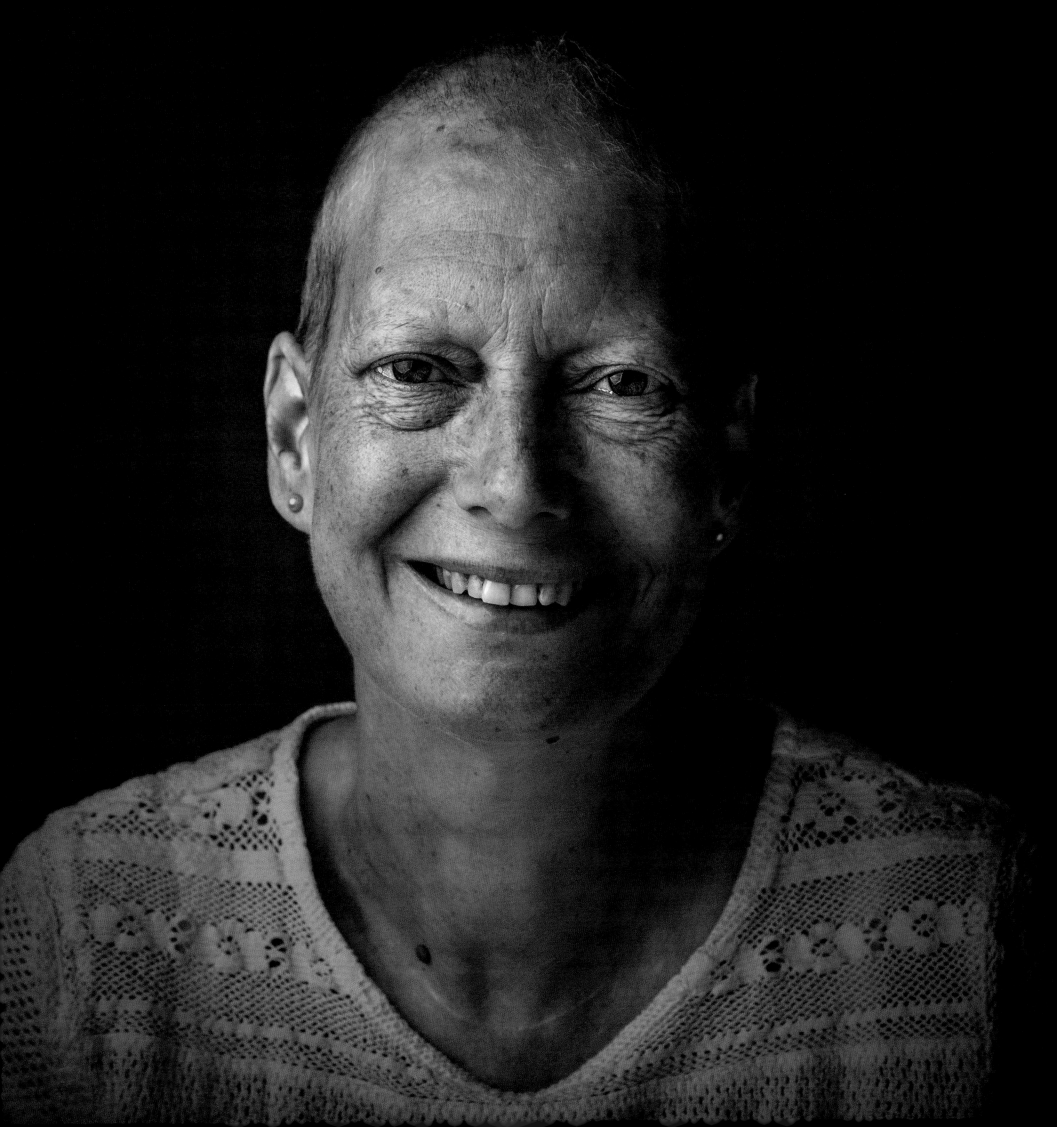

Jo

My story is probably the same as thousands of women, I consider myself relatively healthy, don't smoke, don't drink too much (well not every night!), and I was feeling fine. Breast Cancer certainly wasn't on the cards or part of my life plan but it sneakily decided to take up residence on the muscle behind my left breast!

Last Year in May 2017, at the age of 42 I was diagnosed with Grade 2 Breast Cancer.

I remember the day like it was yesterday, the bombshell that was dropped from a great height. The disbelief and shock of being told you have Cancer, that godforsaken evil word that no one ever wants to hear.

The fear and terror it creates, the uncertainty and unknown path that lies ahead of you. Why me? That is a question no-one can answer.

After numerous appointments of being tested, prodded and poked my journey began with 6 sessions of Chemotherapy, an experience I wouldn't want to repeat in a hurry! Although, I embraced the fact that I was going to loose my hair, I took control and shaved it all off - I wasn't going to let Cancer control me! I considered it a bonus, not having to style my hair every day, I saved a fortune on shampoo!

After my chemo I was scheduled for surgery and just before Christmas 2017 I had a Bilateral Mastectomy and Lymph Node clearance on my left side. For me this was the easy part - getting rid of 'Colin' as the tumour was now known!! Many women fear loosing their breast and find it hard to deal with, no longer feeling feminine. I on the other hand felt nothing towards my breasts; 6 years pervious I had undergone a breast reduction, waste of money that turned out to be!! So to be getting rid of my boobs and getting rid of 'Colin'

once and for all was a relief. My boobs may have been attached to me but I certainly wasn't attached to them!!

After plenty of rest and rehabilitation in February 2018 I faced the final hurdle of my Journey - Radiotherapy! 15 sessions of blasting anything that may be left behind!! Thankfully I sailed through this with no major problems and in March 2018 I was discharged from Oncology. Even though I was elated with this news, no more visits to the hospital, just my yearly check ups and my daily dose of Tamoxifen, the reality soon come crashing in - I was now left to go it alone and pick up the pieces. This is the time when the cancer stuff can start to go a bit crazy in your head! Not only are you trying to recover physically but you also have a lot of mental issues to deal with. A lot of people expect you to finish treatment and immediately be back to 'normal', of course that would be lovely but in reality that doesn't happen! I am very fortunate to be surrounded by a wonderful family who's love and support has been amazing, without them and my warped sense of humour! I am sure my journey would have been very different one.

It has been a rollercoaster of a year, I don't quite know where my inner strength and positivity came from but when faced with the reality that you have Cancer, you have to dig deep and pull on those big girl pants! It has been incredibly tough at times, not just mentally but physically, the scars that have been left are not just the visible ones, I may be cancer free but it will always be present in my every day life - I go to bed thinking about it and when I wake its still there even though it is parked at the back of my mind. I consider myself to be very lucky, I am still here to talk about my journey, so many others are faced with worse and that I cannot even begin to imagine. I know its very cliché but you only get one life, live it to the full and have no regrets.

Jo

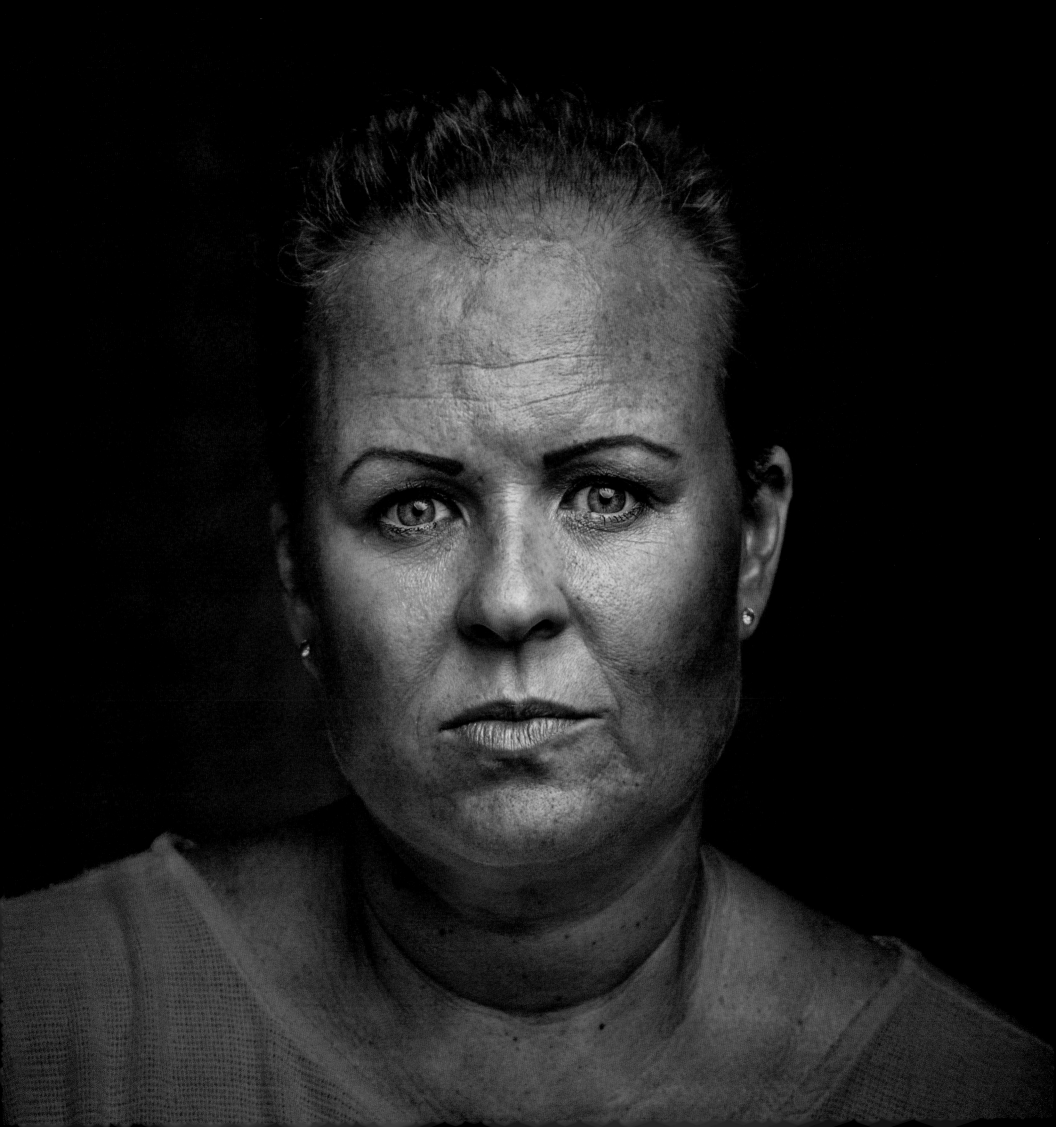

MELISSA

This is my second diagnosis of breast cancer in the right breast at the age of 47. My first was at the age of 36 when my two children were aged 8 and 3 years.

I had a tiny grade 1 tumour and the surgical procedure was a lumpectomy with sentinel node biopsy, three weeks of radiotherapy, Zoladex implants for two years as I was pre-menopausal, and Tamoxifen for five years.

It felt almost shameful to say that I had been treated for breast cancer when other women go through such traumatic experiences.

Once the treatment was over I got back on with life but there hasn't been a day in the last 11 years when I haven't thought about my breast cancer, but those feelings have lessened as the years moved on, with each five years being a major milestone.

Upon receiving a second diagnosis the emotions have been different and I learned from my previous experience that it is a lot easier to be the person with cancer than the people around you who look in and are helpless. Being in that position is far scarier and I certainly wouldn't change places! My Consultant Surgeon has reviewed me annually for 11 years and I imagine it was as difficult for him to deliver the bad news as it was for me to receive it; he is after all human!

The following day I just cried and cried until there was nothing left. There are only two ways to go; further down and give up or fight, and fighting was exactly what I was going to do. I lay in bed and all I could see was a big mountain and a very daunting climb that I wasn't sure I could do but I didn't feel scared this time or guilty and I am not angry.

My family have been amazing throughout this journey and my true friends are those who have remained with me through both breast cancer journeys and I feel no resentment to those who felt they couldn't; that is not my failing.

The treatment plan this time was as I expected so I had already prepared myself mentally for the journey beginning with a mastectomy with axillary node clearance as the cancer had spread to the nodes, followed by chemotherapy, 3 weeks of radiotherapy, Zoladex implants for at least 2 years or until I have definitely gone through the menopause and Letrozole for 10 years.

Chemotherapy has been the most challenging part of this journey, as it not only affects you physically but emotionally and mentally. Cancer is a private illness until you have chemotherapy when it becomes very public due to the visible side effects such as hair loss; but never at any stage of my treatment have I not felt beautiful. Beauty is within you but you just have to try harder to radiate this so people can see it.

I wasn't going to be brave with this second diagnosis; I was going to accept the help and support being offered. I've realised that I'm a much stronger person than I believed I was but I owe that to my Breast Care Nurse who phoned me regularly and was always there for me.

I want to 'own' my breast cancer and use as the motivator to re-evaluate my life and what is important to me. However the journey doesn't end when treatment finishes, which is perhaps the way friends and family see it, and that normal life resumes once again. It moves to a new chapter; perhaps a new me but nonetheless it's on my timescale and my terms. Cancer and treatment has taught me how to be a bit more selfish and put myself first and foremost which has been a difficult lesson to learn!

Melissa

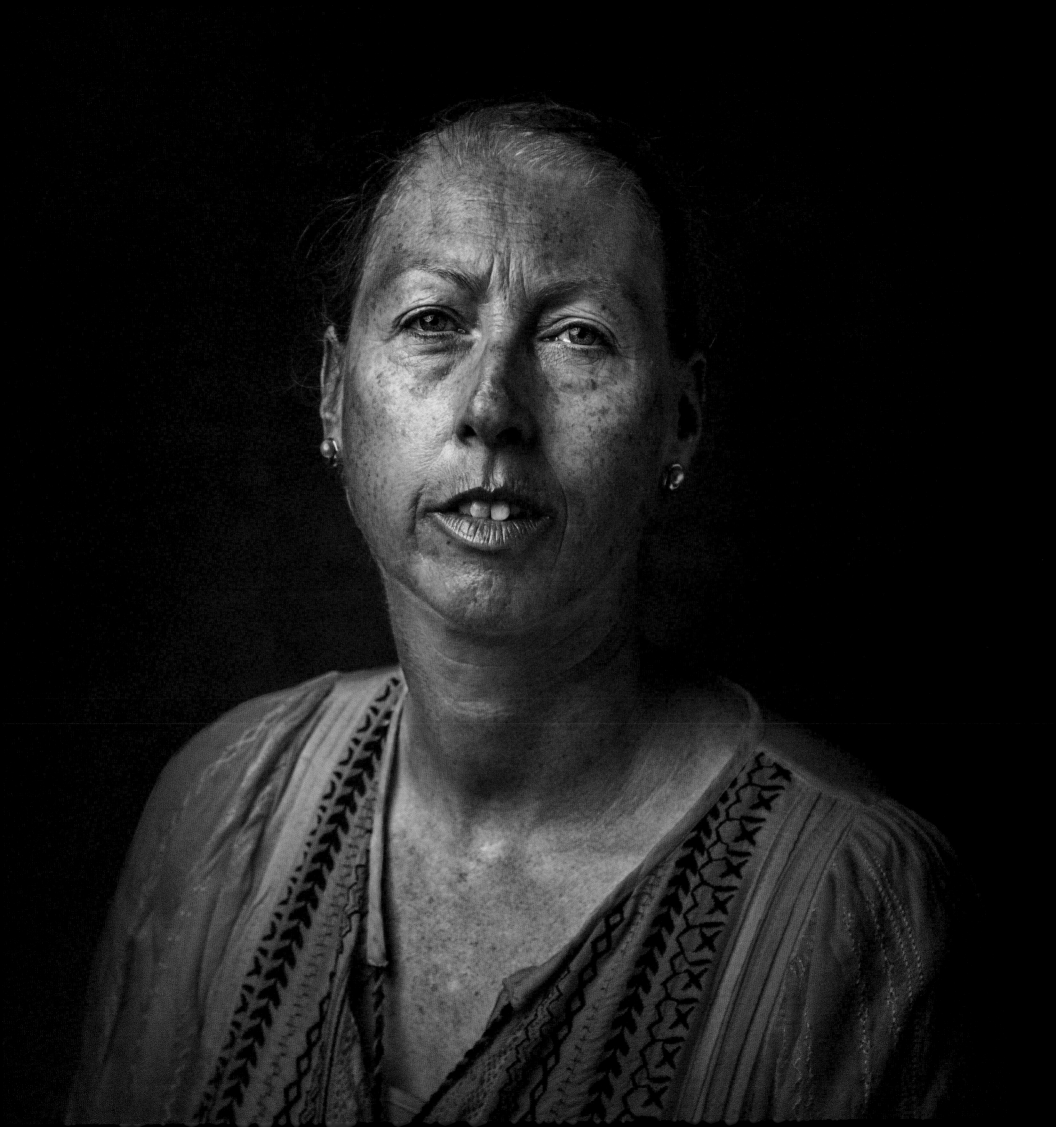

TRACEY

19th April 2017. A day I will never forget. When I got told 'its triple negative breast cancer', all sorts of thoughts went through my head – how, why me, I'm going to die, fear, what about my family, husband and children.

The next few weeks were a blur of appointments and scans, it all felt so surreal. I was just wishing they had got it wrong.

How do I tell my children, was a question I kept asking. How do you tell a 7 and 9 year old their mum has cancer?

I am so proud of how well they took it, their strength and their resilience. We shed lots of tears and tried to spin all the negatives into positives. Along the way although it may seem strange to someone who has not gone through this experience, we also had lots of laughter. A few memories include the time my daughters told me 'I would look like a minion with no hair'. My youngest asking if' I would keep my fringe when I lost my hair' and when asking my eldest daughter to do something she said 'ok mum keep your hair on', this was just after I had lost my hair. I not sure who laughed the most. Laughter is definitely a good medicine.

Chemotherapy started and waiting to lose my hair was hard. In a strange way I couldn't wait for it to fall out as that was one step forward of this journey and hopefully my children would get used to it and still love me.

Chemotherapy was followed by a lumpectomy and lymph node clearance as the cancer had spread to my lymph nodes. Although I suffered some side effects from chemotherapy, I also felt lucky that I didn't suffer as badly as some people do. I think I just prepared myself for the worst. Keeping a positive attitude certainly helped me through.

Radiotherapy followed and then I was offered further chemotherapy as a preventative as there is a higher risk of reoccurrence with my cancer. June 2018 and I had my last chemotherapy.

I was now cancer free. I should have been excited, happy and celebrating but all I felt was fear, all the 'what ifs' going round my head. I have found it a harder since finishing treatment than I thought. Now 4 months since finishing treatment I am slowly trying to get my life back on track, its going to take time but hopefully I will be a stronger person and I have met some amazing new friends on this journey.

I can only advise anyone else going through this journey to stay positive, get support, cry if you want to, laugh if you want to, and although it may not feel like it at the time, there is a light at the end of tunnel.

Tracey

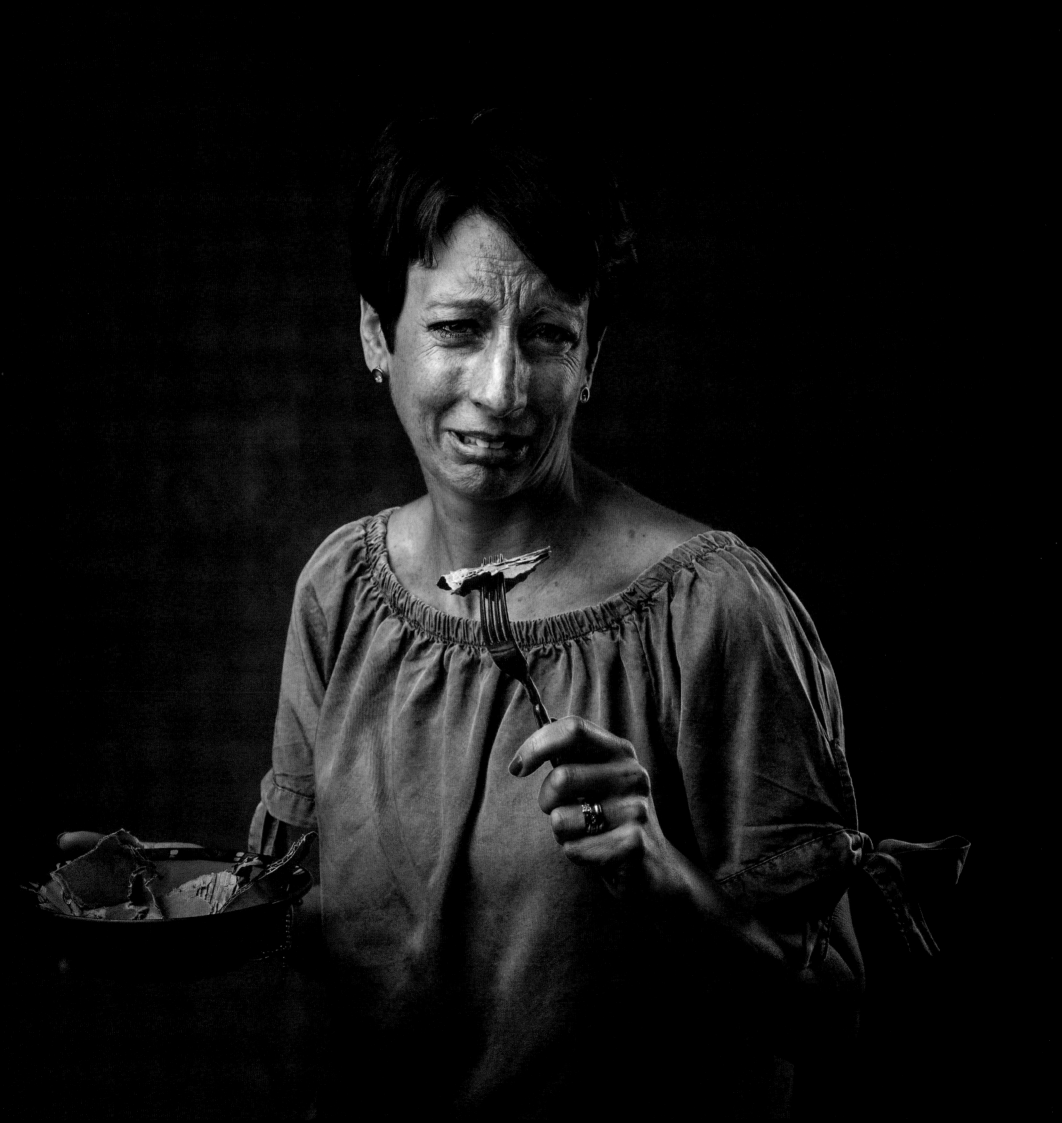

SUE

When I was 31 I never expected to hear the words "It's probably breast cancer... Is that what you were expecting to hear today?"

No, I wasn't! I was young, fit, healthy and just started a new job. In an instant almost everything changed with those words.

Having cancer in my early 30s was initially very lonely and scary. None of my friends knew what to say and my family was distraught. I was suddenly 'the girl with cancer' and I felt so alone. Treatment started. Suddenly my hair fell out and I piled on ten pounds. I didn't recognise the person in the mirror any more.

Luckily I was put in touch with a local group that supports young people with cancer. I met people who just got what I was going through, who I wasn't worried about filtering what I was saying because they had either been through it or were going through it with me. I wasn't the only bald person in the room, I wasn't the only person bursting into flames with hot flushes, I was surrounded by young people like me with cancer and that helped so much.

Whilst I would never, ever say I was glad to get breast cancer, a lot of good has come from my diagnosis. I feel like I'm living a better life now; I don't take things for granted and most importantly I look after me more. I've met some amazing, inspiring people who have helped me through and made life long friends. I try to live in the moment more and appreciate the smaller things. Sounds a cliche I know but it's true. In many ways I'm so much happier than I was before cancer, though the nagging feeling that it might come back will never go away and I still see a stranger in the mirror and in pictures. But, slowly but surely, I'm getting used to the post cancer me.

Sue

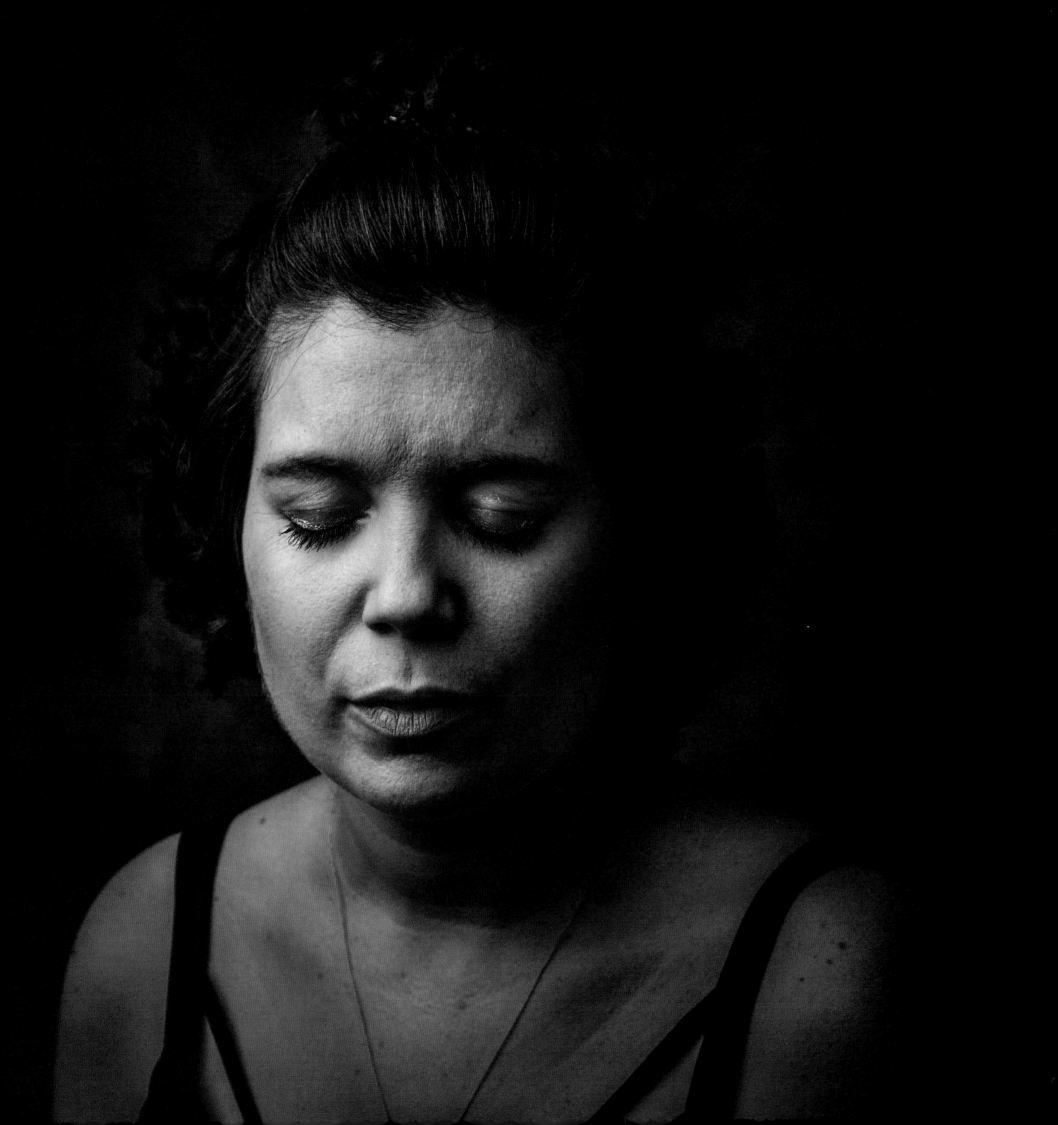

ENCARNI

...and cancer arrives and takes away the everyday joy,

and you keep saying to yourself 'I miss the ordinary problems of day to day living'.

But there is a light at the end when you emerge stronger, wiser and incredibly grateful.

And it is then when you really appreciate the air that you breathe and the hugs of your son.

Encarni

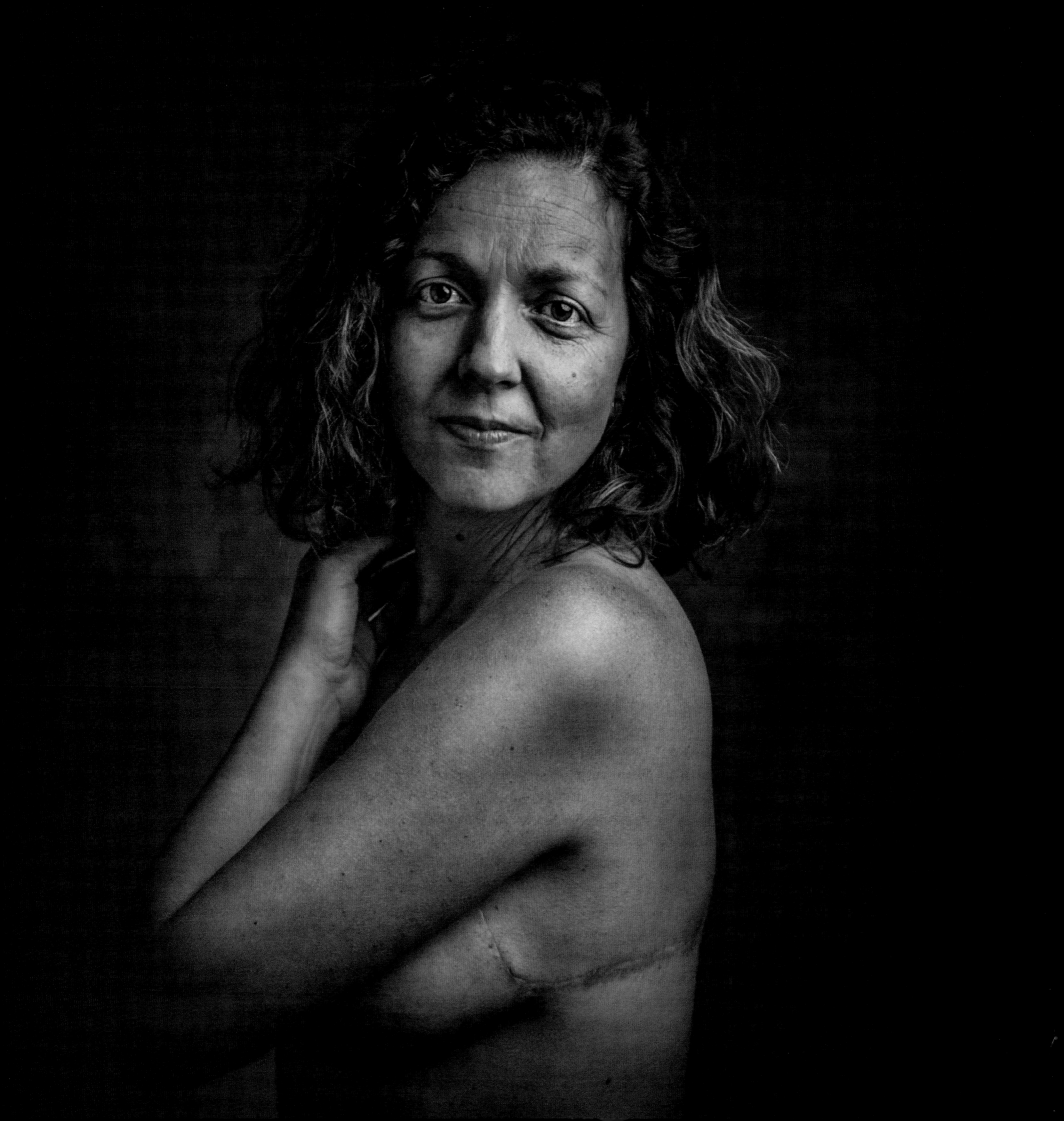

SCOTT

From the initial diagnosis Scott wasn't shocked. He had already been through the process before with oesophagus cancer. After being told it was inoperable and terminal he just asked "How long?". His response was just to shrug his shoulders as if he knew.

Each day in hospital his frustration grew as he just wanted to be at home. He didn't want people to treat him differently, he didn't want to be a burden and tried to be as independent as possible for as long as possible.

He mentioned about going to Switzerland where euthanasia is legal, but laughed eventually when he realised his passport had expired!

He just kept saying "Why me?".

When he reached the end of the four months he was annoyed, he thought he should be gone.

He had numerous infections throughout the last couple of months of his life but was focusing on hoping to spend his last couple of weeks in The Hospice and expressing his wishes about not wanting to end up in hospital.

He went through some spells where he was angry, mainly because he was almost fed up with too many visitors. He felt he needed space sometimes just to be alone.

Loosing his voice near the end frustrated him more than anything, as communication was becoming much harder. But, his smile and thumbs up were enough to let people know he was fine.

Even through his fight near the end he would still say " Don't worry about me, I will be OK! "

Graham and Julie

Sadly Scott died before he could write his story to accompany his photo, so this was written by his close friends Julie & Graham.

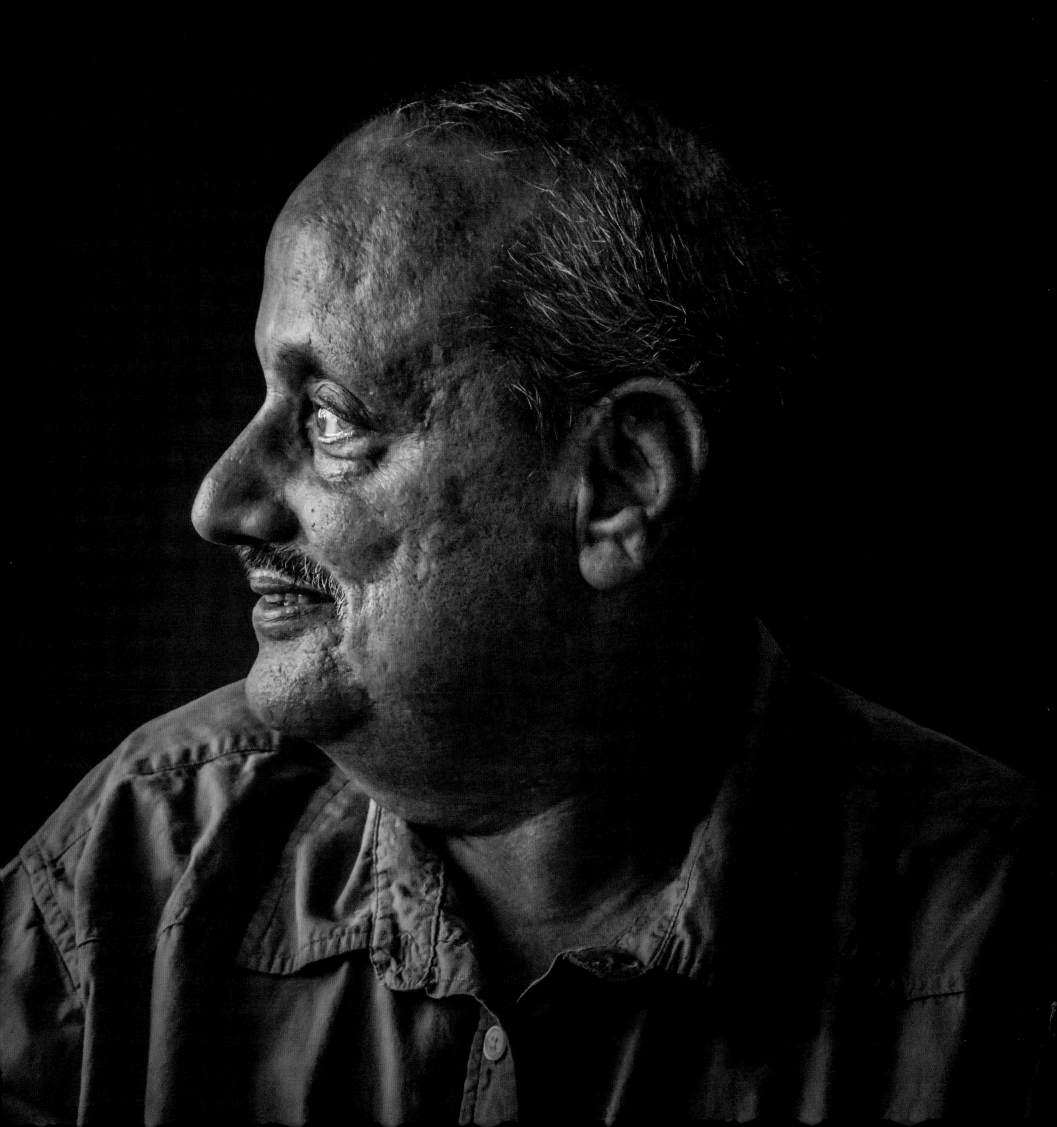

USEFUL LINKS:

www.photographybyimelda.co.uk

www.themonster-series.com/

www.breastcancerkent.org.uk

www.cancerresearchuk.org

www.worldwidecancerresearch.org

www.macmillan.org.uk

www.medicaldetectiondogs.org.uk

A percentage of the proceeds of the sale of this book will be donated to the following charities:
- Breast Cancer Kent
- Cancer Research UK
- Worldwide Cancer Research